After qualifying as doctor at Barts Hospital, London in 1978, Peter spent 16 years as a rural GP practitioner in Tiptree, Essex.

Seeking new challenges, he spent the next two years in Western Australia working as a flying doctor, mainly in Aboriginal communities.

On returning to the UK, he gained a commission in the Royal Navy as a surgeon commander which included various postings in Europe, and deployments to Afghanistan, Malawi and the Gambia.

He became the last serving ship's doctor on HMS Ark Royal aircraft carrier before the ship was decommissioned in 2011, followed by several years as a medical repatriation doctor visiting 50+ countries.

What has evolved is an interesting 'journey in life' and many stories need to be shared, some amusing, many life-changing, many very unusual, but mostly rewarding for his patients and him.

I dedicate this book to my children, James and Celine, and all my grandchildren, who have lived and endured many of the memorable moments in this book.

**Peter Fowler**

# TAKE A SEAT

Journey in Life as a GP

AUSTIN MACAULEY PUBLISHERS™
LONDON · CAMBRIDGE · NEW YORK · SHARJAH

Copyright © Peter Fowler 2023

The right of Peter Fowler to be identified as author of this work has been asserted by the author in accordance with sections 77 and 78 of the Copyright, Designs and Patents Act 1988.

All rights reserved. No part of this publication may be reproduced, stored in a retrieval system, or transmitted in any form or by any means, electronic, mechanical, photocopying, recording, or otherwise, without the prior permission of the publishers.

Any person who commits any unauthorised act in relation to this publication may be liable to criminal prosecution and civil claims for damages.

All of the events in this memoir are true to the best of author's memory. The views expressed in this memoir are solely those of the author.

A CIP catalogue record for this title is available from the British Library.

ISBN 9781398467644 (Paperback)
ISBN 9781398467668 (ePub e-book)
ISBN 9781398467651 (Audiobook)

www.austinmacauley.com

First Published 2023
Austin Macauley Publishers Ltd ®
1 Canada Square
Canary Wharf
London
E14 5AA

Without the advice, support and encouragement from my biology teacher, Mair, at the Sir Henry Floyd School in Aylesbury, I would have never considered even applying to study medicine but as a result of this, I have experienced an amazing 40-year career as a doctor for which I thank her enormously.

I also thank my wife, Sue, for indulging in me joining the Royal Navy at the age of 50, only three years after we were married, at a time of life when most people are contemplating winding down. I only got away with deploying to Afghanistan for three months by buying her a six week around-the-world business airline ticket to meet friends in Canada, Argentina, Australia, New Zealand and South Africa!

I am forever grateful to Surgeon Commodore (Rtd) Paul Hughes, whom I first met when I was considering joining the Royal Navy. His advice and encouragement greatly helped my many enjoyable years within the service.

# Table of Contents

| | |
|---|---|
| Introduction | 11 |
| Why Don't You Apply to Study Medicine? | 14 |
| 1979–1983: House Jobs/GP Training | 30 |
| 1983–1998: General Practice | 43 |
| 1999–2000: Western Australia | 67 |
| 2000–2004: Back Home – What next? | 111 |
| 2004: Commissioning into the Royal Navy | 115 |
| 2004–2012: Royal Navy Medical Officer | 130 |
| 2004–2019: International Medical Repatriation Doctor | 165 |
| 2018: Time to Start Winding Down | 180 |

# Introduction

Peter Fowler was born in Aylesbury, Buckinghamshire in 1954. His father died when he was very young so growing up was quite hard especially as his mum never remarried. He was educated at the Sir Henry Floyd Grammar school in Aylesbury and then went on to study medicine at St Bartholomew's Hospital, part of the University of London. Thankfully in those days, university fees and expenses were paid for by local authorities, otherwise the rest of this book wouldn't have happened.

He completed his medical degrees in 1978 and then started four years of training at Stoke Manadeville Hospital and Oxford to qualify as a general practitioner (GP). From 1983–1998, he worked as a GP in a semi-rural practice near Colchester in Essex.

Having got divorced during this time, Peter decided that it was time for a 'Life change' so in 1998, he accepted a post as a locum GP working for the Western Australian Centre for Remote and Rural Medicine (WACRRM). This proved to be an amazing two-year experience, working in a variety of GP practices and hospitals throughout the state (The size of Western Europe) along with time with the Royal Australian Flying Doctor and remote Aboriginal Health services.

On returning to the UK in 2000, it was really crunch time as to where to go from here. After a few months working as a locum, he joined a private GP practice in the city of London where he worked for the next three years.

It was now 2004 and he was 50 years old. By pure chance, an advert appeared in some of the medical journals that summer advertising for experienced doctors to join the Royal Navy. Assuming that 50 years old would be considered a bit too old, he cheekily applied. After an informal 'Acquaint' visit to the dockyards at Portsmouth, he was put forward for Officer Selection and Commissioning. Soon after, he attended the rigorous three-day Admiralty Interview Board (AIB) and was offered a commission. This was followed shortly afterwards by six months of intensive 'Militarisation' including a term at the Britannia Royal Navy College (BRNC) Dartmouth, where he passed out as a surgeon lieutenant commander.

Peter spent the next eight years as a commissioned naval officer, being promoted to surgeon commander after his second year in service. Over the coming years, he served in Cyprus, Gibraltar, Italy, Afghanistan, Malawi and the Gambia, culminating in 12 months as ship's surgeon on the Royal Navy's Flag Ship, HMS ARK ROYAL, visiting Canada, USA and Germany.

Peter left the Navy in 2012, then spent his remaining time as a GP working for the military at various bases throughout the UK but as a civilian medical practitioner (CMP) rather than uniformed. He also became quite active working for an International medical repatriation organisation helping to escort sick and injured people from all over the world back to the UK. At the last count, he had undertaken 189 of these from more than 50 different countries, all successfully.

At the age of 65 and after 40 years practising as a doctor, Peter retired. There are many personal anecdotes he wanted to record. Read on.

# Why Don't You Apply to Study Medicine?

At 11 years old, I passed the entrance examinations to attend a grammar school. I was accepted at the Sir Henry Floyd School in Aylesbury, Buckinghamshire. This was a co-ed school. I enjoyed my time there and gained 12 'O' levels. When I was 17 years old, I had an interest in joining the RAF as a pilot. I went down to the Officers and Aircrew Selection Centre at RAF Biggin Hill airfield for a three-day aptitude test which involved multiple written papers and interviews, culminating in a simulation of flying a jet. In reality, it was actually a big cardboard box with knobs and levers. At my final interview, the wing commander indicated that I wasn't suitable for pilot training but they might consider me to train as a navigator. Bugger that I thought. I wanted to be in the front of the jet not in the back. That was the last thought I gave to joining the military. When I chose my 'A' level subjects, I had no idea what I wanted to do career wise. It had been assumed by my teachers and indeed my mother that I would go to university as my elder brother had done. He was four years older than me and had originally applied to study medicine but didn't get a place, so did a BSc in biology instead. He then went into advertising! We were estranged for over 30 years through no fault of ourselves (That's another story). We finally met up unexpectantly at our mother's funeral (Co-ordinated by my ex-wife). This prompted a further get together during which we tried to fill in all the many gaps in our separated lives, then he died suddenly in his early 60s of a pulmonary embolus before we could rekindle our relationship.

I was not particularly arts nor science orientated at school and hence chose subjects that I most enjoyed, namely biology, geography and British constitution (Basically English Politics). This caused rather a stir in the school as the teachers had to arrange me an individual timetable that crossed both the arts and sciences faculties. I was the only student to do this at that time.

I'd always been interested in anthropology, geology and archaeology and thought that I would end up studying one of these subjects at university, perhaps to train as a teacher. However, during the lower sixth form, my biology teacher, Mair, suggested that I should consider applying to medical school. Nobody had ever previously become a doctor from my grammar school and certainly not from my family.

I did not think at this time that I was anyway bright enough to become a doctor and there was just one other stumbling block, I was studying a rather diverse mix of 'A' levels. However, after further enquiries, I discovered that some medical schools admitted students with 'Non-science' backgrounds, provided that they do an initial year (Much like a foundation degree course) called $1^{st}$ MB, equivalent to 'A' levels in biology, chemistry and physics, most of the subjects I had been trying to avoid! If successful with this, the formal five-year medical degree would then start.

When the time came around, I duly sent off my five medical school preferences. I included St Bartholomew's Hospital in London (Barts) as Mair, my biology teacher, had contacts there and knew that it had a very good reputation. I added another London teaching hospital and three provincial universities.

After what seemed like a lifetime, the brown envelopes started arriving in the post. Rejection, rejection, rejection. Manchester offered me a place with three-grade A 'A' levels. Rather optimistic I thought. Finally, the last letter arrived. It was obviously from Barts but having had basically four no, what hope in hell was there of an offer. Low and behold, I was invited for an interview. What would they ask me? Nobody in my family had ever worked in the medical world. I'd had chickenpox, scarlatina and had my adenoids and tonsils out as a child but this hardly made me an authority on medicine. On my application, I had mentioned that I'd represented my school at sport (I came $2^{nd}$ in the county school's triple jump one year and was a fair tennis player but I hated cricket, football and rugby). I'd also been in the Scouts throughout my school years and achieved the Chief Scout's Award. All in all, though, not an outstanding CV.

Thankfully, the interview went quite well with no questions such as: "How would you perform a quadruple heart bypass?" or "Discuss the functioning of the adrenal glands?" To my utter amazement, a couple of weeks later, a letter came in the post offering me a place to start $1^{st}$ MB at Barts if I achieved 'An average' of two-grade C 'A' levels. Can you imagine nowadays being accepted to medical school with two C's?

It was the summer of 1972. After sitting my 'A' levels, my mother and I flew over to Ottawa in Canada to see my aunt, uncle and cousin. When we returned home, my 'A' level results were waiting. Was it all going to be a distant dream?

Biology-Grade B, Geography-Grade B, British Constitution-Grade B.

I'd done it! With only a few weeks to find accommodation in London and a whole library of textbooks to buy, there was no time to lose. What had I let myself in for? In six years, I would hopefully be a doctor! Being quite late receiving an offer from Barts, I could not get into the student's hall of residence in Charterhouse Square (Just off Smithfield Meat market) and eventually through the student union accommodation unit was offered a room in a house in Tulse Hill, South London, not ideal as it involved quite a long overland train journey into Blackfriars station then a brisk walk to the college in Charterhouse. I went to have a look at the room before moving in. The room was dark and cold. I was assured that it would be redecorated before my arrival. The owner of the property was a stern, grey-haired woman who only ever wore black and who looked like Cruella DeVil out of 101 Dalmatians. Her husband was bed-bound and actually died whilst I was lodging there. They had a maniac unemployed son who kept wanting to be mates. I moved in, wallpaper still hanging off. There was an electric meter on the wall of my room which seemed to guzzle 10p coins like no tomorrow and always seemed to cut out just as I was trying to do some late-night homework for the next day. Breakfast was served punctually at 7 am, dinner at 6 pm. The only consolation was that there were two other fellow students also going to be at Barts (David and David) for whom I remain eternally grateful in helping me with my physics and chemistry homework every Sunday evening after returning from home to this hovel.

On day one at the college, the Dean addressed us all. We were an eclectic bunch. There was John H, previously a radiographer, John F, who previously worked in a bank, Brian G, a former accountant and Andrew S, a psychologist, all several years my senior and then me, a fresh-faced 18-year-old straight from school. The Dean tried to reassure us that the hardest part of becoming a doctor was securing a place at medical school but as the next six years was to prove, there would be plenty more hurdles yet.

$1^{st}$ MB was a tough year and there was the constant threat that we would be thrown out of the college if we failed the final exams. Against this was the fact that by now in my mother's eyes, I was already practically a doctor. I have since looked back at some of the original exam papers from this time and have no idea how I passed them. Sheer will power and hard grafting I suspect.

Passing $1^{st}$ MB felt like a huge relief. Next term, we would be starting $2^{nd}$ MB, an intensive two years of 'Pre-clinical' training. Unlike many of the newer medical schools at that time, there was no contact whatsoever with 'Live' patients during this phase.

$2^{nd}$ MB was made up of anatomy, physiology, pharmacology and biochemistry, although all quite detached from anything really human. This was the time that we each purchased a 'Half skeleton' from the college (I recall they cost about £100 even then in 1973). These were genuine human bones unlike today when they are usually synthetic. Heaven knows where they all came from. They came in their own wooden boxes, a bit like a small coffin. Imagine dropping it on the floor of a bus or train and seeing an array of human bones scatter amongst the crowds.

Anatomy involved groups of 6–8 students each having a dedicated cadaver on which we spent two years dissecting down to the bone, learning the course of every nerve, blood vessel and structure of every organ. I remember that first day when we all piled into the anatomy department, a really cold, dark and scary Victorian building in Charterhouse Square. We were allocated to our corpses shrouded in smelly formalin sheets. Then, an anatomy demonstrator (Usually a trainee surgeon) pulled back the cover to reveal what for most of us was our first view of a dead person. When I look back, we were never given surgical gloves to perform these grisly tasks and it often took days for the smell of death and formalin to dissipate from our hands. What made anatomy worse was the fact that we were examined weekly on what we had learnt at each practical session and if only one of us failed, the whole group failed. This meant hours during evenings memorising muscle origins, nerve pathways and bony structures in preparation for the next examination.

Bearing in mind that I had tried avoiding anything to do with chemistry during my school life, Biochemistry was even more of a mystery. On day one, we were budded up and told that we would be spending the whole day analysing our own urine pH, testing specific gravity, salt content etc, etc. John F was supposed to be my buddy and I was banking on him knowing a lot more about the subject than I. But John F didn't appear. I later found out that he had broken his leg playing football and would not be starting the course for another week or so. Poor John had to contend with my woeful mark from my solo effort.

The final component of $2^{nd}$ MB was physiology from which at least we could start to understand the relevance of science to actual human functioning. Many a teaching session centred around live but anaesthetised animals and how they reacted to the application of various chemicals and drugs. I doubt that anything like this still occurs in medical schools because of the animal welfare issues and also nowadays 'Models' can now be made which look very lifelike (Look at the operations seen in the TV series Holby).Somehow, I got through $2^{nd}$ MB and had a well-deserved summer break before the three years 'Clinical' when we would finally be allowed to see real, live patients. By the time we had purchased our starched white coat and Littmann stethoscope, we were almost there!

Throughout the clinical period, we continued to have regular daily lectures and practical teaching but were also assigned to different specialities or 'Firms' to gain hands-on practical experience. At the cornerstone of all patient contacts was learning how to take a full medical history from the patient, examining them and then trying to figure out what on earth might be wrong with them. This initially seemed a complete mystery, most likely because we had all spent the previous three years with no live patient contact whatsoever. Many a patient was so used to being used as a guinea pig on the ward that they would verbally take us through the whole process, even telling us what investigations they should have. Days were very full of lecture after lecture, demonstration after demonstration, then pounding the wards for that vital patient hands-on experience. We were required to sign in for every lecture. I have to admit that there were days when we'd had a heavy drinking session the night before and not turn up but we had a backup agreement that our mates would sign us in instead. This worked OK until the lecturer declared that on one day, Joe Bloggs had been signed in six times for the same lecture.

At each lecture, we would try and scribble down as many facts and figures as we could. There were very few handouts, no computers and most presentations were done with handwritten overhead acetates. As a result, by the end of three years clinical, I had accumulated a ton of paperwork on all those presentations. What was supposed to act as the basis of my final exam revision proved pretty worthless as most of them appeared unreadable, superfluous and non-sensical. So, it was back to the textbooks. At least these were succinct and clear, especially the revision exam hot topic books.

Time was so tight that often we had to snatch our lunchtime sandwiches whilst watching the pathologist doing autopsies (Post-mortems) in a grand timbered galleried theatre. As the pathologist triumphantly lifted an organ onto the waiting scales, he declared with glee, "And this liver breaks the record for being the heaviest this term!" I'm sure he'd have won 'Britain's got talent' with his act.

My introduction to cardiology was somewhat soured when 3–4 of us medical students attended our first cardiology clinic. We were thrown an ECG recording by the consultant (Which none of us had ever seen before) who then barked, "And what does this ECG show?" None of us had any idea. "Get out of my clinic and don't come back until you do know."

As a result, none of us ever did go back. So much for guiding and mentoring one's students.

Thankfully, I learnt how to read an ECG at a later occasion.

On the subject of cardiology, on one occasion I got the chance to go into an operating theatre to observe a heart bypass. As one could imagine, this was quite gory at close quarters; blood pumping through loads of tubing everywhere. That evening full of excitement on my eventful day, I went over to my girlfriend's house for supper. Her mum proudly came into the dining room and announced that we were having stuffed hearts! As I viewed these organs on the plate, I couldn't help but see them as another anatomy lesson. "Doesn't the left ventricle look odd when it's cooked!" I retreated from the room feeling extremely nauseous. I don't think my future parents-in-law were too impressed.

We had to do two attachments in obstetrics and gynaecology. Unfortunately, there were few and far between baby deliveries at Barts itself and those that did occur were usually snapped up by young aspiring registrars who needed to get their tally up. As a result, I spent a month at the Northampton maternity unit for one of my obstetric stints. Talk about a production line, I had it off to a tee so well that I'd be going from delivery room to delivery room teasing the little blighters out before I'd even had a chance to introduce myself to the aspiring mother. As I recall, I must have delivered over 35 babies whilst there.

There was a distinct lack of interest in general practice (GP) training within the medical school. It was pretty well ingrained into us from an early stage of 'Clinical' that Barts was a centre of excellence in cardiology and neurosurgery and that we should all be aspiring to be the next top neurosurgeon or Christian Barnard, taking on heart transplants. There was not even a department of GP at this time, although in later years this was rectified and they even appointed a professor of GP. As a result, we were told to organise our own GP attachments if we felt so inclined (So much for a rounded balanced view of medicine). I'm quite sure that some of my contemporaries didn't take up this chance and used this time as an extra few weeks holiday. In the end, I contacted my family GP practice back in Aylesbury who readily took me on, sitting in during consultations and doing home visits together. It would be these opportunities that would spur me on to choose general practice as my career choice later on. Interestingly, over half my year of students subsequently went on to further GP training after qualifying. I'm sure the college must have felt that it had failed in its remit.

Neurology (The study of diseases of the nervous system) seemed a complete mystery. Having spent two years intimately dissecting a human body, it didn't make understanding this speciality any better. The professor of neurology always prided himself by stating that he could usually make a firm medical diagnosis of the patient merely by asking 3–4 questions and these were usually the patient's name, age and occupation. Any examination only added the icing to the cake. He used to parade his patients in front of us medical students onto a stage in a lecture theatre and delight in making us all look like idiots from our sparse knowledge of the subject. Some would be limping, some with a tremor, others a stammer. One favourite of his was to get a student down to the front of the class to demonstrate to all how to examine the 12 cranial nerves. The trick here was to immerse oneself head down frantically writing notes so as not to be picked out, as the slightest eye contact with him would be our downfall and certain embarrassment. To this day, even though no longer working, I still walk around and try to spot diagnose people's ailments. "He's got Parkinson's" or "He's had a stroke".

One of the highlights of 'Clinical' was the opportunity to go away and study paediatrics at a hospital abroad for three months as an elective. We were given a list of potential placements and I was lucky enough to be accepted to join the Monmouth Medical Centre in New Jersey, USA. I wasn't sure how I was going to fund this adventure since I was being supported purely by my local authority back in Aylesbury in addition to any pocket money earned from holiday jobs. Over the college years, these included being a Schweppes drinks production line worker (Which put me off ever drinking tonic water again) and a hospital ward orderly. I remember working as a casual postman over a couple of Christmas periods but got taken aside several times by some of the regulars as I was completing the deliveries too quickly and showing them up. I was told sternly that I should go home for a couple of hours once I'd finished my rounds before returning to the sorting office to pick up the next drop. I also worked in an East End pub just up from Barts occasionally. This could have easily been the set for 'Only Fools and Horses'. It was real sawdust on the floor place but I got cash in hand with a free meal thrown in so well worth it. I was taught by the owner how they inflated the price of drink rounds as the night went on and the pundits became more inebriated. This went hand in hand with 'Recycling' all the beer dregs from the trays back into glasses for re-sale. There seemed to be a lot of dodgy dealings at the bar with 'Delboy' lookalikes wearing gold bling and sheep's skin coats handling huge wads of money. I don't think that I would walk back from that pub to my digs alone at midnight nowadays.

Thankfully, I didn't resort to another source of income that many of my contemporaries did through much of the clinical phase that is supporting the 'Wank bank' in Harley Street. At £5 a throw, this was quite a lucrative earner at that time and helped as beer money.

My concerns about the elective proved unnecessary since the sponsor of this particular attachment was a rich American businessman who financed eight Barts medical students a year. Not only did we get our return flights paid for but we were put up in the Princeton University club in New York City for 3–4 days after we arrived (All expenses paid). Once at the family ranch in New Jersey, we had the sole use of a huge 4x4 truck, all food included, and our own wing of the house and even a generous weekly allowance slipped into a small brown envelope under our pillow by our housekeeper. In fact, I returned home with more money in my pocket than I'd gone out with.

The most significant aspect of the US system of medicine I witnessed was the discrimination between those who had and those who didn't, which often incorporated the way coloured patients were treated. This even involved separate entrances to different units within the hospital. One of the most bizarre things I saw here was the day when the paediatric team were required to go and collect a new-born child in an incubator from another hospital. The ambulance turned up and apart from the two paramedics, four doctors including myself jumped on. Immediately, they started sounding the siren and flashing the blue lights and off we rushed. After about 30 minutes, I noticed that we were slowing down, and then we completely stopped (Blue light still flashing). At this point, one of the paramedics opened the back door and asked who wanted a Big Mac. Yes, we had driven into a Drive-through! We then casually proceeded to collect our patient.

Another amusing incident was when I was following around on a paediatric ward round. The consultant was surrounded by what looked like about 12 junior doctors. There was a prolonged discussion about the clinical presentation and results of all the tests for one of the children. It culminated in the consultant saying, "Yes, I think we have an FLK."

After the ward round, I went up to one of the Interns and asked what an FLK was. "We get a lot of these," she replied. "Funny looking kids."

I can't say I learnt much about paediatrics during my three months but I certainly got to see a lot of the Eastern seaboard of the US and even a week up in Ottawa with some relatives!

About the same time as I was in the US, a couple of my contemporaries did a similar elective to Cape Town. Christian Barnard's theatre scrub boots adorned the student's bar at Barts for some time afterwards.

As Finals quickly approached, there was an air of total panic as we all realised that after six years at medical school our futures depended entirely on passing the final examinations. We were now being tested on all the knowledge and skills we had hopefully learnt in medicine, surgery, obstetrics, gynaecology, pharmacology, paediatrics, ENT, psychiatry and dermatology. Over the course of several weeks, we would have to write dozens of essays, answer numerous multiple-choice papers and sit through a number of oral vivas. Everything depended on these exams as there were no summative assessments at this time.

It was very disconcerting that in previous years, quite a number of students had failed one or more of the final examinations which meant them having to spend a further term at the college prepping to re-sit (And potentially losing their first hospital post as a result). Because of this, a large number of us sat and passed another qualifying exam in the run-ups to finals known as MRCS and LRCP (Member of the Royal College of Surgeons and Licentiate of the Royal College of Physicians). This not only served to be an excellent way to revise for degree finals proper but it meant that we went into the examinations already fully qualified as a doctor and entitled to use the title 'Dr' which was an obvious feeling of achievement.

Despite six long years at medical school, I came away feeling honoured and privileged to have had the opportunity to study there.

The history of Barts remains so intriguing when one considers that the first hospital was established in 1123. It is the oldest hospital in London and the oldest hospital in Britain still providing medical services on the site it was originally built on.

Most early hospitals offered little more than rest; a good diet and spiritual comfort until the fifteenth century. Outside the hospital, illness was explained by a complex set of ideas that merged religion, magic and folklore. In the 1530s–50s, Henry VIII disbanded monasteries, priories and convents (The Dissolution of the Monasteries). This act left Barts as a hospital in a precarious position by removing its income. However, King Henry VIII refounded the hospital in 1546, and signed an agreement granting the hospital to the Corporation of London.

The magnificent Henry VIII gate incorporating a statute of the king above the archway was built in 1702. It is the only such statue in a public place in London.

Barts was at the forefront of medical developments including the work of William Harvey who conducted research on the circulatory system in the seventeenth century whilst Percival Pott and John Abernethy developed important principles of modern surgery in the eighteenth century.

Historians have suggested that students first attended St Bartholomew's in 1662. By the 1880s, St Bart's had established itself as the largest medical school in London. It was also here that some of the current day developments in nursing were advanced in the late nineteenth century.

The hospital was rebuilt between 1730–1759. In the remaining North Wing, lies the magnificent Great Hall, a Grade one listed building approached by a grand staircase, the Hogarth Stair, which the English painter, William Hogarth, painted. At the west end of the Great Hall is a striking portrait of Henry VIII, hands on hips and glaring down at all who enter. A combination of the mystery of the stairway and the ever-watching gaze of this most belligerent of monarchs makes this a suitably intimidating arena in which to examine final year medical students. I know because I was one of them!

In 1993, the controversial Tomlinson Review of London Hospitals was published and concluded that there were too many hospitals in central London. It recommended that the service should be delivered closer to where people lived. Barts was identified as a hospital with a catchment area that had a low population and the hospital was threatened with closure. A determined campaign was mounted to save the hospital by the 'Save Barts Campaign'. Some facilities were saved but some like A&E services were moved to other hospitals.

St Bartholomew's Medical College was subsequently merged along with the Royal London Hospital Medical College into Queen Mary and Westfield College in 1995.

# 1979–1983: House Jobs/GP Training

It was now late 1978. Finally, I had the initials MB, BS, MRCS, LRCP after my name and I was a fully-fledged doctor. What would the next 40 years have in store?

The next big event was to get married in January 1979. During my undergraduate years, I had done some holiday work as a Theatre Orderly at Stoke Mandeville Hospital, not far from where I was brought up in Aylesbury in Buckinghamshire. I got to know various consultants during this time and as a result was offered two six-month House Officer (HO) posts in surgery and medicine. There was no submission of a CV, no references or interviews, just a nice chat over coffee. Stoke Mandeville was and still is a renowned spinal injuries unit but was initially founded as a plastic surgery unit for injured pilots, especially burns, during WW2.

My first post as a newly qualified doctor was HO in surgery under a great consultant, Mr McA. We were a small team consisting of the consultant, registrar, SHO and myself, the HO. There were only four surgical teams in the hospital at that time and we rotated a 1:4 on-call roster for acute surgical admissions and a 1:2 on-call for two surgical teams for routine out of hours duties. There was no European working directive in these days and our daily work was done when it was done, even if it meant being on the wards or in theatre all hours of the day and night. My job was to clerk in new admissions, arrange appropriate investigations and prep patients for surgery.

The wards at Stoke Mandeville Hospital were of the original WW2 Florence Nightingale style, large long single-story wooden buildings with a row of beds down each side and perhaps a couple of single rooms. The sexes were completely segregated to different wards. Each ward was run by an experienced ward sister/matron who even the most distinguished consultant feared. Ward rounds each morning could only commence once sister was entirely happy that everything was 100% in shape. Patients would be sat up for inspection in their perfectly made beds, colourful arrays of flowers adorning the bedside tables. The doors to the ward would then be ceremoniously opened to allow the entourage to enter.

When on-call for admissions, we would admit patients straight in to the ward as there were no Surgical Admissions Units at this time. On one occasion, a local GP had requested that we take a young Indian lady with acute abdominal pain, likely appendicitis he had assumed. She arrived on the ward and even on cursory examination, it was obvious that she was a nearly full-term pregnancy and was actually in labour. She apparently had no idea she was pregnant. After a spontaneous normal delivery, I was thankful for my previous 30+ deliveries as a medical student. It was quite apparent that her GP could not have even examined her.

Another young girl came in with a likely appendicitis, and having scrubbed up with my registrar on numerous occasions before, he offered me the chance to perform the operation under supervision. As I made my incisions through the skin, muscle and peritoneum in her right groin, a gush of dark blood spewed out. This was no appendicitis. It was a ruptured ectopic pregnancy. We got the Gynae registrar over to remove her fallopian tube and as if any consolation, I removed her appendix.

I recall one evening sitting at the nurse's station on a ward completing my notes. I overheard two nurses trying to coax a little old lady to walk down the long ward. "Come on, Mrs Jones, just a few more steps."

"I can't go any further," she replied.

I looked up only to see that her ever stretched bladder catheter was not only attached to her but also still attached to the side of her bed several metres away. For a moment I had a Benny Hill moment envisaging her catapulting back along with the ward should the nurses release their hold.

My consultant was an excellent all-round surgeon and on any surgical list, we could be doing a bowel resection for cancer, thyroidectomy, mastectomy or even a limb amputation. I could never however get too excited peering into another opened up abdomen even if my boss became ecstatic when he discovered the 'Best gallstone' he'd ever seen or the biggest prostate he'd removed. Amputations were always hard to deal with. I think my consultant realised my distaste which is why he probably always handed me the severed limb to ceremoniously carry into the sluice room.

We seemed to undertake a lot of sigmoidoscopes in the clinic. This is when a long cold metal pipe-like instrument is passed up the rectum to look for causes of bleeding or tumours (No fibre-optics in these days). I recall on one occasion a chap was duly lying in the 'Foetal' position naked on the couch ready for some cold steel. I entered the cubicle with my consultant who squealed, "Is that the famous hunt scene I've heard about?" Sure enough, the whole of the patient's back was completely tattooed with colourful huntsmen and hounds.

"But where's the fox?" asked Mr McC.

The patient sniggered, parted his buttocks to reveal a fox's tail disappearing into his anus! "Gone to ground," he replied.

On another occasion, a rather attractive 30+ year old lady also came into clinic requiring a sigmoidoscopy. She was advised to remove her 'Bottom bits' and adopt the familiar 'Foetal' position. We pulled back the curtains to be greeted by a very curvaceous totally naked woman wearing only knee-length leather boots. "Will that do?" she asked.

"That will do very nicely," my consultant whispered as he approached her rear end.

As a house officer, we were the first doctor to take a patient's medical history and perform an examination before presenting the details to the consultant for further assessment. One particular old lady was admitted with a variety of symptoms indicative of cancer-anaemia, weight loss, and abdominal pain. I felt very sorry for the old dear and didn't want to poke her about too much as she looked so frail. When the consultant finally came around, I presented my findings feeling quite chuffed with myself.

"So where is the primary cancer?" he enquired.

I said that I'd not found anything suspicious.

"Any masses in her breasts?" he replied. But I hadn't examined her breasts as she was a frail old lady. When the consultant lifted up her nightgown, there was a huge craggy ulcerated tumour on one of her breasts. I would never make the same mistake again.

Although I thoroughly enjoyed my six months of surgery, it made me realise that I had no inclinations to pursue a surgical career.

This job was followed by six months as a Medical HO under another great mentor, Dr C. He had a keen interest in liver and gastrointestinal disease and as a result, I became quite adept at performing liver biopsies (But not with the benefit of ultrasound guidance like today). I subsequently taught many a new registrar my newfound skills. This post was, as expected, much more ward-based, organising blood tests, X-rays and scans. Again, after six months, this was not to be a career changer.

At the time of doing this job, my then wife was training to be a beauty therapist and was fascinated about plastic surgery. I had got to know one of the consultant plastic surgeons quite well and during one discussion he asked if my wife would like to see him perform a facelift. We duly went over to his private clinic one weekend. I say clinic but it was more like a spare room in his detached house. Anyway, in came the lady who proceeded to sit on the reclining couch. The surgeon started drawing lines all over her face, forehead and neck. After scrubbing up, he proceeded to inject local anaesthetic around all these lines. Yes, he was going to do a facelift under local. He started incising around her face to the point one could almost lift it all off, at the same time as having a normal conversation with the lady. Well, at this point, my wife blacked out cold, thankfully away from the patient but nonetheless still very embarrassing. We had to make our exit swiftly and never again did I suggest anything similar.

I was pretty much set on becoming a GP during my year as a houseman. Luckily, Stoke Mandeville had a well-established GP Vocational Training scheme (GPVTS) in collaboration with the John Radcliffe Hospital in Oxford. Having been working at the hospital for a year, after discussion with the GPVTS organisers and some decent references from my two consultants, I was offered a place. This would involve another two years at the hospital as a 'Senior' House Officer (SHO) covering core GP specialities (Paediatrics, obstetrics and gynaecology, ENT, A&E, geriatrics and psychiatry) followed by 12 months in a GP training practice. One of the main reasons that I chose this scheme was that my local authority in Aylesbury had fully sponsored me financially throughout medical school and I felt that as a token of appreciation, I could give something back to the local community.

The six months post in paediatrics involved three months on a general children's ward and three months in the special care baby unit (SCBU) which involved looking after premature and sick babies. Although SCBU was fascinating and enjoyable, I wonder how much its real value was in regard to training to be a GP.

During a paediatric ward round on one occasion, we got to the bed of a young Asian girl probably about eight years old. She was sitting up in bed with her neck and back arched and her jaw in spasm. She had been fully investigated and no obvious underlying cause was found. It was even being mooted that her symptoms were all psychological. Whilst the consultant was deliberating with his staff, a new locum paediatric registrar happened to walk past the entourage and quite casually said, "Nice case of TETANUS in bed 10." It was only then that the penny dropped and everyone realised that this girl was displaying all the classical although rarely seen symptoms of Tetanus. Thankfully, despite the delay in reaching a diagnosis, she made a full recovery.

Obstetrics could be quite scary because one was always dealing with two potential patients. Over my three months in this job, I became very proficient at doing forceps and Ventous vacuum-assisted vaginal deliveries, although when you see such interventions, they look very unsavoury. I was on the labour ward one day when an Asian woman was brought in by ambulance obviously in the advanced stages of labour. It didn't help that she could not speak English and this was before the days of routine availability of translators. To cap it all, the baby was in a breech position meaning bottom not headfirst. Very few babies are born breech nowadays as the risk of brain damage is increased because of the head being the last thing to deliver. However, she was too far on to organise even an emergency caesarean section so my registrar decided that we would have to go ahead with a manual delivery. We followed all the guidelines and successfully delivered a healthy baby bottom first.

20 years later, I received a formal-looking envelope enclosing a letter from a firm of solicitors asking me to confirm whether the name they supplied was me. It transpired that the parents of this baby I had helped deliver all those years before were suing the health authority with whom I'd been employed, as the child had subsequently developed some mental and physical handicap. The reason for the very long delay was that any claims had to be submitted before the

21st birthday of the claimant. Having confirmed my involvement in this case I then had to wait several months to find out what the outcome of the investigation was going to be. Luckily, as I was always trained, writing good clear medical notes is very important. On this occasion, they were perfect. Thankfully, I eventually received another letter stating that all my actions had been thorough and professional and that no further actions were to be taken. However, I had had to endure months of uncertainty and stress.

I can't think to imagine how many 'Bimanual' examinations I did during my gynaecology attachment. This is where one examines the pelvis with one hand pressing down on the lower abdomen whilst the other hand examines vaginally. On one occasion I was doing a joint clinic with my consultant. He had done a bimanual examination and was obviously impressed by the size of the lady's uterus. "This is a good one to feel," he said to me. "Have a feel and see what you think," with no consideration for the poor lady who was about to have a second prodding.

I must say that I found it very difficult to accurately determine the size of a uterus, after all, what could one compare it to. We were subsequently taught to compare the size of the uterus to different stages of pregnancy, e.g. the uterus is just palpable above the pelvic bone at about 12 weeks' gestation and at the level of the umbilicus at 20 weeks. Eventually, I grasped how to assess uterine size and then could at least confidently tell my consultant, "This is a 16-week sized uterus, sir."

"Well done, Fowler," he replied.

The very same consultant could be quite abrupt and verbally aggressive to others. On one particular ward round, which I always dreaded for this very reason, we were all standing around a patient's bed. I gave him a brief outline of the patient's presentation and examination.

He then asked me what her HB (Anaemia test) level was. I scoured her notes and just couldn't find it recorded. At that point, he lashed out, called me incompetent then kicked me quite hard on the shin, enough to make me reel. "Now go and get it," he snarled. I somehow think that this sort of behaviour nowadays would result in disciplinary action especially as he acted like this with an audience present.

A&E was hard work. In these days (1981) there were no A&E consultants, and most of the time, the department was manned by people like me, usually alone. There were no such things as medical or surgical assessment units. The role of the A&E SHO was to either deal with the problem at hand or call in the appropriate specialist doctor, whether it be medical, surgical or orthopaedic. I recall several occasions when we would be on duty alone in A&E for 36-hour stints, often covering 09:00 on a Saturday until 21:00 on Sunday. We were lucky to get an hour or two's sleep in the early hours of Sunday morning once all the drunks and head injuries had cleared. Nowadays when you walk into an A&E department, there are doctors everywhere and all have consultant emergency staff 24/7.

One hears nowadays that A&E departments are inundated with trivial minor health problems which shouldn't be there at all but we did get to see some quite unusual presentations.

One evening, a chap in his 20s, arrived in the department with his mother. As Mum recited, poor Nigel had blacked out in the bathroom and when he woke up, the toilet brush had miraculously disappeared up his rectum (Bristles first). Sure enough, one could just feel the tip of the plastic handle high inside his rear end. From my reading, this appears not to be an unusual reason for attendances at A&E. Poor chap had to have a general anaesthetic to retrieve the offending object. Not sure if we returned it to him! Mum didn't sound at all surprised or perturbed.

On another occasion, another young man attended stating that he had lacerated his anus. How one might ask could this have happened. Well, he was walking along a riverbank, claimed to have slipped and a bulrush just happened to penetrate his rectum. As it does!

Another evening, a chap turned up in A&E with a very lacerated scrotum. The story given was that he had been sitting alone in a bar then started chatting to another guy who invited him up to his flat for a 'Nightcap'. When he finally realised that there was more to this encounter than he'd envisaged, he tried to escape through the sash window which fell and shattered on him traumatising his genitals. Well, that's what he told me!

Then there was the nun in her full regalia who attended complaining of a vaginal discharge. One felt a bit uncomfortable asking a nun to disrobe for an internal examination but she appeared quite relaxed about it. We soon found the culprit for her symptoms as I removed the screw cap of a coke bottle from the roof of her vagina. I haven't drunk coke since!

During my three months psychiatry posting, I worked mainly in a geriatric unit. The building itself was a dull red brick Victorian establishment with all the characteristics of the 1975 film *One Flew Over the Cuckoo's Nest*. Many of the in-patients were severely chronically depressed, others had bipolar disorders. Bedside discussions with most patients were impractical as many were mute. I had the unenviable job of conducting the weekly ECT (Electroconvulsive therapy) clinic. This is a procedure done under general anaesthetic in which small electric currents are passed through the brain, intentionally triggering a brief seizure. The theory is that ECT seems to cause changes in brain chemistry that can quickly reverse symptoms of certain mental health conditions. I'd perhaps do about six of these per session. The patients would expressionlessly shuttle from the ward to the ECT room whereby one by one they would be laid on a couch, the anaesthetist would place a rubber guard into their mouth, gas them to sleep, and then I would give the electric shock. I was never convinced of seeing any substantial improvement in these poor individuals but I gather that the practice is still performed around the world.

Finally, it was time to start the year in proper general practice. I had been allocated to a lovely rural practice in Haddenham on the Oxfordshire/Buckinghamshire border. My trainer, Jonathan, was a really enthusiastic GP and he eased me into what would become the art of general practice by us doing joint consultations and home visits. One day a week, all the GP registrars attended a day release scheme either at Stoke Mandeville or the John Radcliffe in Oxford. Here we would be introduced to the likes of Balint, Neighbour, Pendleton and Schofield, all quite innovative doctors at their time and all of whom had studied the doctor-patient relationship as a partnership rather than "Me doctor, you're only the patient, so do as I say!" (As I would soon find out in my forthcoming new practice, no one had told the patients that they were in a partnership). On a humbling note, I had the opportunity to meet and treat my childhood GP who happened to have retired in the village where I was working.

The senior partner was a great character. A very wisely GP with nothing too much trouble to help. He had a call one night to go and do a home visit. To make the point about appropriate use of services at unsocial hours, he went in his flannelette pyjamas, dressing gown and slippers.

On one occasion, my trainer asked me to go and visit a lady who had requested a home visit, the story being that she couldn't leave the house because of D&V. On arrival, I knocked on the door; she answered and let me in. She was very young and extremely attractive. I suggested that I ought to feel her abdomen to make sure there was nothing too acute so we both went upstairs to her bedroom. She laid on the bed and undid her dressing gown to reveal skimpy lace knickers and bra with full-length stockings. Just the right attire for someone who's housebound I thought. I completed my examination, reassured her all was well and made my quick escape. I dreaded to think what she would have done had the senior partner turned up wearing his pyjamas.

In the last few months of vocational training, I started to apply for GP partnerships. We looked as far west as Tintagel in Cornwall, Boston in Lincolnshire, a scattering in East Anglia and several within the Oxfordshire/Buckinghamshire area. My wife and I had both grown up in the Home Counties, so we didn't really want to settle anywhere north of the Watford Gap. At this time (1982–83) it was not uncommon for a practice to receive 50–60 applicants for a new partner. How things have changed today where many practices can't attract any new partners at all.

The Tintagel practice was very keen for me to join them to the point that one of the partners drove all the way up to Aylesbury to interview me. I subsequently went down to see the practice in February. My wife was expecting our first child so was reluctant to travel all that way mid-winter, so I travelled alone. I must say driving across Bodmin moor in the middle of winter wasn't pleasant, trees growing at 45 degrees due to the fierce winds. It was very curious that I was not introduced to the second GP partner during my whole two days there. Also, when I was informed that the area was grid-locked by holidaymakers during the summer months but snowed in during the winter, I decided that it was not the practice for me.

I was finally offered a partnership in a semi-rural practice a few miles south of Colchester in Essex but only after my wife and I were subjected to a weekend of 'Trial by sherry'. This involved my wife being whisked off by the other wives, lunches and dinners, whilst staying at the senior partner's house. Driving home after this ordeal, we mulled on the merits of the practice but before we had reached home, one of the partners phoned us to formally offer me a partnership. This was to be the start of 16 years there.

# 1983–1998: General Practice

It was early 1983 when we moved to Essex to take up a position as a GP. I joined as a new fourth partner. We had a practice population of about 10,000. We were constantly busy. We had no computers when I started so everything was handwritten or typed by a secretary. On average each partner saw 40–50 patients a day and we did about six home visits a day each to the elderly and infirm, something rarely undertaken nowadays. Then, on top of this, we were on duty for the practice for out-of-hours medical cover 1:4.

In addition to regular GP work, I was also a part-time lecturer in the department of social science at the University of East Anglia, a clinical assistant in gynaecology, ran a number of local authority family planning clinics and was a GP Trainer, mentoring younger doctors who were in training to become GPs themselves. Between 1990–92, I studied for and gained an MSc in general practice through Guys and St Thomas' hospitals. During 1995–6, I had the desire to do some more studying (Why?) but rather than do more medical courses, studied and gained a diploma of wine qualification.

Being on-call for out of hours was always a bit of a bugbear, as when one's seen so many patients during the day, to then start doing home visits during the night or at a weekend was very tiresome. Over the years, most GPs moved their out-of-hours duties to local doctor-on-call groups. This did however cost quite a bit (It was £5–6,000 per annum per GP when first introduced) and most GPs then had to work on-call shifts to cover the costs or suffer less income. As for myself, I continued to do my regular on-call for the practice for the entire 16 years.

I was always amazed that patients could call the doctor in the middle of the night for anything. One night, the phone rang about 2 am. "Hello," I said, "Dr Fowler here. What can I do for you?"

"I don't want you, I want to speak to Dr M," she replied.

"I'm afraid Dr M doesn't live here with me." Did she actually think that we all slept together? She rang off!

I remember a young girl phoning and waking me about 3am one day demanding emergency (Post-coital) contraception for unprotected sex. When did the accident occur? I asked.

"Five minutes ago," she replied.

"I think we can deal with this at the surgery in the morning," I replied.

Visiting the elderly was nice although quite time-consuming especially as we worked in quite a rural area. I visited one old lady monthly for several years. She always had a dusty old bottle of Emva cream sherry on the sideboard and would pour me a small tot every time I called. On one occasion she said she had a little something to give me. She passed over some crumpled tissue paper and to my horror when I opened it there was a complete set of porcelain dentures.

"My father had these made for me as a 21$^{st}$ birthday present," she said. "I know that you collect medical antiques." They had lasted her over 60 years but she finally invested in a new set as the originals kept falling out when she spoke! I could never face having this set of teeth on display in my antique cabinet.

A rather well-known schizophrenic came in one day clutching a paper bag, saying that he had bought something for me. He too knew that I collected medical antiques and informed me that he had come across an interesting brass surgical instrument. I unwrapped the bag to find that he had given me a garden rose sprayer. At least my wife was happy.

The one exception when a patient came in with something worthwhile was when a chap who worked in the surgical instrument industry came in with an interesting mahogany box under his arm. On opening, there was the most amazing set of surgical instruments including amputation knives, bone saws of every description, skull trephining tools and various other indescribable instruments of torture. All the components were genuine nineteenth century and to think that these were all used before the invention of anaesthetics.

Another of my regular elderly ladies lived with her daughter. She was bed-bound and quite frail.

On one occasion, I visited her as usual and as I left, told her that I was going away on holiday for two weeks but that I would put her down for a follow-up visit on my return. The day I returned to work, one of the receptionists informed me that the lady's daughter had called the surgery and requested that I pop around to see her mum that lunchtime despite the fact that I was not due to visit her for another week. I duly went and we sat and chatted for a while, then she held my hand and said, "Thank you for popping around and thank you for everything you've done for me." This puzzled me. I parted shortly and drove back to the surgery only to be informed that the daughter had called to let me know that Mum had passed away minutes after I had left the house.

Not all deaths were sombre. There was one occasion when I was called to see an old chap who I knew quite well and had collapsed in his garden. When I arrived at the house, there was this dead-looking man lying on his back on the lawn still clutching his watering hose which was spurting out water into the air like some macabre fountain ornament. By now there were half a dozen neighbours peering over the fences, all muttering that George didn't look too well. I eventually managed to get someone to turn off the hose and confirmed George's demise. I called upon the observing neighbours to come and help me move George indoors for some dignity but his wife stated adamantly that she didn't want a dead person in her house! After much deliberation, she saw reason and we managed to manhandle the old chap into the hall to await the undertaker. The funniest part of this incident was the fact that I offered to contact our local funeral director to come and make arrangements. She hesitated then said, "Thank you but I think I'll stay with the co-op, then I can get some dividend stamps."

I was in the surgery doing some paperwork when a call came through from reception requesting that a doctor attend the local co-op store, just across the road from the surgery as an old lady had collapsed. On arrival, I was met by the duty manager and taken into one of the food aisles where there was a very dead-looking lady lying on the floor. Confirming her death, I suggested that we should move her to a more suitable location. The cold room at the back of the store he suggested. For some reason, the manager had not considered closing the store or evacuating the other shoppers despite this inconvenience. So, the manager took the lady's ankles and I grabbed her around the upper chest and we precariously carried her up the aisle towards the back of the store. However, we came across another old lady pushing her shopping trolley who stopped right in front of the frozen peas section blocking our path.

Already feeling knackered from carrying such a dead weight, I politely asked if the lady would move over and let us pass. Without even taking her eyes off the frozen peas, she said, "I was here first, you wait your turn." Thankfully at that point, she turned to see what must have looked like a scene from a Monty Python sketch. We finally got the deceased into the cold room.

At that very point, a delivery man arrived carrying a box of goods and walked right past the corpse without any sense of surprise. "Dead, is she?" he muttered.

Although as doctors, we see a number of deaths over the years, it was always something I found hard to deal with. There was one occasion that I was asked to attend a patient's house as a neighbour had not seen the chap who lived there for several days. By the time I got there, the police were already on the scene, as were several neighbours. We scoured the property. There were no doors unlocked and all the windows were tightly shut. The police decided to break a window in the kitchen door to get in. The key was still in the door. They unlocked the door, pushed it open and entered the kitchen. There was then that fearful thought of where he might be, what injuries he might have. Was he dead? We searched every room thoroughly, even every wardrobe, under every bed. Nothing. No body. But the house was locked up from the inside. Having all decided that perhaps no gruesome deed had been done, we re-grouped in the kitchen. As we left the house, one of the policemen went to close the kitchen door only to find that there was another door immediately behind it. On opening this, there was our man, crouched on the WC, probably having died several days previously. What an undignified way to end one's life.

On a happier note, I will never forget a lady in her late 80s who was always immaculate in her dress, smart hair, painted nails and the rest. I used to visit her husband regularly who had very advanced dementia. She found it very difficult to cope given that he was prone to verbal and physical abuse. After 50 or so years married, they could no longer sleep in the same bed as he thought of her as a stranger. Then one day he passed away. I didn't see her again for several months until she arrived at the surgery, arm in arm with a 40 something year old man. I inquired as to what I could do for them. "I just wanted to know if I'm fit enough to have sex with this young man," she replied.

"You certainly are," I responded. Her face lit up. They left grinning like Cheshire cats. That was the last I saw her.

Despite dealing on a daily basis with patients' ailments and tales of woe, there were many lighter-hearted moments. One day a middle-aged lady came in saying that she was due her cervical smear test. She declined having a chaperone. I pulled the screen across the couch and asked her to take her bottom bits off and pop onto the couch. I checked that she was ready then pulled the curtain aside only to see a complete full-length artificial limb propped up against the wall.

Without even thinking, I just said, "You didn't need to take your leg off." Then made the situation even worse by saying, "Right, we'll just do the smear then. Could you part your legs, sorry leg?" Luckily, she did find it quite amusing.

In my training, we had always been encouraged to take a holistic approach to patients care. This caught me out however when a lady came in with a sore throat. I dealt with that then said, "Whilst you're here, why don't we just check your blood pressure." (Me thinking I was going the extra mile) I applied the BP cuff to her right arm and pumped it up waiting for the dial to give me her BP. Nothing happened. I removed the cuff and reapplied it again. Same outcome.

I apologised to the patient, now feeling rather incompetent.

"Don't worry," she replied. "A lot of people don't realise that I've got an artificial arm."

Another lady came in with a sore throat. I checked her over and felt she could be managed with symptomatic treatment only. She seemed happy with my advice. Scanning her medical records, I noticed that she was overdue for her cervical smear. "Shall we just do your smear now while you're here?" (My holistic approach again). She obliged and left shortly afterwards.

At coffee break, one of my staff called me aside. Mrs S had just returned to reception and bleated out to all and sundry, "That young doctor's a bit too keen. I only went in with a sore throat and by the time he'd finished, I'd had a smear test."

Many a time, patients commented on how young I looked. I knew when time was taking its toll on me several years on when one old lady said to me, "Didn't you used to be the young doctor?"

My wife at the time used to suggest what clothing attire I should wear as I was never really that bothered. Bearing in mind this was the early 80s, I had no hesitation in going to work in white trousers and loud stripy boating jackets. On one occasion, I did a home visit to an old lady. As she opened the front door, I announced that I was the doctor.

She just looked me up and down and said, "You look more like a tennis player!" I mellowed my dress after this. At least my dress sense didn't reach the heights of one of my partners who had a penchant for pastel-coloured safari suits which he had originally worn whilst working in Fiji as a young doctor.

One of my special interests as a GP was family planning and sexual health. I recall a lady in her 30s who came in for a routine cervical smear test. Thankfully, this patient had both her legs. I couldn't help but notice a tattoo across her pubic region. I couldn't quite make it out. "What does the tattoo say?" I asked.

"It says DAVE," she replied.

"When did you get that done?" I asked.

"When I was about 18," she replied.

"Hasn't it caused any problems over the years having DAVE embossed over your privates?"

"None at all," she said, "as I only ever go out with guys called Dave."

I'll always remember an attractive young girl coming into the clinic requesting her repeat Depo-Provera contraceptive injection. Like most women, she declined a chaperone (Although nowadays we as doctors would be strongly advised to insist if only to protect ourselves from any accusations). I offered her the choice of having the jab either in the upper arm or buttock. She chose the latter. I pulled the screens across and asked her to expose her buttock for the deed. As I pulled the screen back, there she was leaning over the couch, skirt on the floor, wearing the smallest thong I'd ever seen. She turned her head over her shoulder towards me and said, "And how do you want me, Doctor?" Perhaps I should have had the chaperone after all!

In one of the family planning clinics I worked in, my female colleague and I were asked to see a couple who had been unsuccessful in conceiving. She was a gigantic obese woman; he was a short skinny guy. They had been through a whole series of infertility investigations all of which had been normal. At their last outpatient review at the fertility clinic, a locum doctor felt quite baffled as to why they hadn't managed to conceive. He asked them to describe how they had sex and then it all became apparent when for the last five years, the little man had been sticking his penis into her tummy button. As sexual health counsellors, my female colleague and I were tasked with trying to teach this couple the art of normal sexual activities. For an hour a week over 6–8 weeks, we saw the couple and gave them exercises to practice. No joy! They thanked us very much for our time and then requested that we refer them for IVF.

I worked with some great nurses in the family planning clinics. One of them was asked to give a presentation on contraception to a group of female schoolteachers. Halfway through the talk she produced a number of rubber penises from her bag and lined them up on the table. They were an assortment of sizes, shapes and colours. She then asked them all to pick a penis on which to demonstrate the application of a condom. That would have been an interesting 'Fly on the wall' picture to witness.

The same nurse had a group of teenage boys come into the clinic wanting some 'Johnnies'. She realised that there was a lot of bravado within the group. She got her box of condoms out of the drawer and asked them whether they wanted small, medium or large. That flummoxed them.

Amongst the many odd consultations I did, I was always surprised when a woman would come in just to ask me how she would know if she'd had an orgasm. My response was usually, "You'll know alright".

An awful number of women don't know what a circumcision is and trying to explain it to someone in lay terms was quite difficult. It might have been easier to just drop my pants and show them!

On one occasion, one of my wife's girlfriends came in saying that she was due a cervical smear. I wondered why she had chosen me rather than one of the other partners. Only a week or so before, she and her husband had been around our house for dinner. She popped up on the couch, legs akimbo. As I was peering up her nether region performing her smear, she quite calmly said, "That was a lovely dinner party the other day!" I didn't dare tell my wife. Several months late, the same girl came in again complaining of some shortness of breath and a dry cough. Her chest sounded clear and with her known history of allergies, I started her on a steroid inhaler. She returned after a couple of weeks feeling much better. I felt pleased with myself until one of my partners came in another week or so after and informed me that she had been back to see him with weight loss and night sweats. A chest X-ray revealed Non-Hodgkin's Lymphoma. This was treated successfully and she made a full recovery. And, she even came around for dinner subsequently.

I knew that the time was coming when I should stop performing cervical smears as it got to the stage that I had to get reading glasses and whenever I bent down to perform the act, found that they had either misted up or at worse fallen off. Bit of a problem when one's wearing sterile gloves and manipulating a vaginal speculum!

Moving on swiftly from the nether regions to breasts. A young girl came in one day concerned about a breast lump. She declined a chaperone, so I pulled the curtains across in front of the couch and asked her to remove her top bits for an examination. I examined her as I'd been taught and reassured her that everything was quite normal. As she was re-dressing, she enquired whether that was the standard method of examining breasts. I didn't quite understand why she had asked. It only transpired that the last time she had a similar examination whilst living in London, she had been seated in the surgery, the doctor had asked her to unbutton her blouse, stood behind her and had then examined her breasts from inside her bra. What could I say?

For some time I was the youngest partner in the practice, the other three GPs all being several years my elder. We were all chatting one day and I just happened to say how surprised I was that so many young girls came into the surgery obviously anticipating a chest examination either because of a chesty cough or breast symptoms but who were not wearing a bra. I assumed that this was the norm until all three partners almost in unison declared that it never happened to them!

When Caverject (One of the first drugs to treat male impotence) was initially released, the drug rep came around to the surgery to explain this amazing breakthrough, its giving technique and mode of action. The rep was a young attractive girl and when she produced a large rubber penis from her briefcase, I wondered how many times a day she fondled these demonstrators. Even now I find it difficult to see who would want to self-inject this drug into their own penis. Anyway, equipped with a couple of free samples, my day came when a tubby old diabetic chap came in with his wife to discuss his impotence. "I've just the thing for you," I said. "All you have to do is stick this needle into the shaft of your penis, inject the solution, give it all a bit of a rub and bobs your uncle."

"But I haven't even seen my penis for the last five years," he replied.

"Don't worry," I replied, "we'll get your wife to do it."

"I'm not going anywhere near it," she retorted.

I never had a chance to experiment on anyone else and what a relief when Viagra came on board.

Because of my interest in family planning, I was approached by the respective medical pharmaceutical companies for the then new implantable female contraceptive, Norplant, and the first drug eluding intrauterine device, Mirena. On behalf of these companies (And for a token financial offering) I went around to a number of GPs to demonstrate their respective fitting techniques. This proved quite lucrative as I supervised some 500, which was until some problems started appearing with the implant. There was a surge in numbers of women who wanted them subsequently removed but few doctors trained in this procedure. So, there I was, going around to all these GP surgeries again to show them (At a small fee again). The most memorable occasion was when I was asked to show a senior consultant gynaecologist how to remove one of the implants on a private patient on whom he was going to perform sterilisation. Normally, I would use a simple pair of specially designed forceps and a scalpel on a normal surgery couch. On this occasion, I was escorted into a huge operating theatre at a private hospital, fully scrubbed up and gowned and presented with a whole major surgery trolley of surgical instruments. I felt a bit awkward merely picking up a couple of items to use!

As you can imagine, over the years we as GPs had a lot of contact with funeral directors none more so than a local chap who was a builder by trade and undertaker in his spare time. He was always very efficient and collected the deceased very punctually. At this time if a body was to be cremated, it required two independent doctors to certify that there were no suspicious circumstances before the death certificate could be issued. Our friendly undertaker had a makeshift barn in his back garden in which he kept the bodies in black zip-up body bags on trolleys prior to disposal. The worse part about doing the cremation certificates was the fact that we often had to let ourselves into the barn when the light was low, identify 'Our' body, unzip the bag and do a cursory examination of the corpse, ensuring that there were no obvious knives sticking out or ligatures around the neck. For our troubles, we received a small cash payment which was always known as 'Ash cash' discreetly placed in a brown envelope on the trolley.

One day, I was out on a house call, my wife was at home and the doorbell rang. On opening the door, she was confronted by our very same funeral director, a gaunt pale-looking man dressed in a black long-tailed coat and top hat. In the drive was his big black hearse complete with a coffin. "Is this Dr Fowler's house?" he enquired. My wife looked petrified. "I'm glad I found the right place. Could you give him this envelope when he gets home?" One can imagine what my wife was like when I got home.

I've always had an aversion to feet (I'm glad I didn't train to become a chiropodist). They seem to be a part of the body that a lot of people ignore. I recall a grubby old farmer coming into see me as he'd noticed a small lump on one of his feet. He took his shoe and sock off saying, "I washed it this morning especially for you."

*Thank goodness*, I thought. I wasn't quite sure what this lump was so asked him to remove his other shoe and sock so that I could compare each side. He looked up in horror.

"I didn't wash that foot."

On another occasion, I was asked to call around to see another farmer at home. He opened the hall front door and I was instantly puzzled why he was wearing wellington boots. As I stepped into the hallway, I felt a recurrent squelch with each footstep and it was only then that I noticed about a dozen hens and ducks happily wandering around the furniture.

It was a similar story when I was asked to go and visit a couple of old spinsters. They were both ex-actresses and extremely eccentric. They spent most of their life in bed upstairs arguing. The only problem was that their only WC was off the back of the kitchen. When I arrived, I entered the hall and proceeded upstairs to meet them. I couldn't initially understand why my feet were making a squelchy sound until I noticed that the carpet was soaking wet, and then it twigged. The poor WC obviously didn't get much usage.

One of my most notable diagnoses as a GP was on a chap who had been with the practice for several years. He was huge, 6'5" tall, with a chisel jaw and hands like a giant. I had trained at St Barts hospital in London and they had a very famous endocrinology department which we as students would frequent as there were sights there one would never see elsewhere. This chap reminded me of a case of Acromegaly where the pituitary gland overproduces growth hormone to produce in effect, Giants. Remembering this, I quizzed my tall man and to my surprise, he stated that he had had to buy bigger and bigger hats, gloves and shoes over the recent years (Which is a feature of excessive production of growth hormone but he hadn't considered this abnormal). I duly referred him to the professor of endocrinology at Barts where my diagnosis was confirmed and not long afterwards, he underwent removal of the pituitary tumour. He would obviously remain a giant for the rest of his life but at least I saved him some future expense buying bigger and bigger clothing and not least the risk of a premature death. I must say that my GP partners were a little miffed at my clinical prowess.

"My bowel has fallen out," was the response from an elderly lady on the phone one day I was on duty.

*Just another normal day,* I thought. Arriving at the patient's house, there was no response to ringing the doorbell so I let myself in through the kitchen door calling out her name. I could hear a few grunts from the hallway. I was quite shocked to find this very old lady propped up against the hall table and sure enough her entire small intestine was in a pile between her legs. I don't know why but the medical school never seemed to teach us how to manage a 'Bowels on the floor' scenario. All my instinct told me to do was to wrap the bowel up in a moist towel to try and minimise any shock. The hardest thing following this was to convince 999 that I needed an ambulance ASAP. Even when the ambulance crew arrived there was a certain, "Oh right, Doc, so her bowels have fallen out, ha, ha, ha." They had a different expression on their faces when I removed the towel to reveal the mess on the floor. Amazingly, the patient underwent surgery to replace her bowel and repair her ruptured vaginal wall and made a full recovery.

As a GP, one can never appear surprised or shocked by a patient's presentation such as the oriental patient who came in to see me with a chesty cough. I suggested that we have a listen to his chest. On exposure, I noticed a number of curious circular bruises over both the front and back of his chest. I racked my brain trying to figure out what these could be. Then he told me that he'd been to a traditional Chinese therapist who had performed 'Hot cupping' to try and treat his cough. Traditionally, cupping supporters believed that the intervention removed harmful substances and toxins from the body to promote healing. According to the British Cupping Society (Which I only recently discovered even existed) cupping therapy can be used to treat rheumatic disorders, fertility problems and even varicose veins. I think my patient elected to try a course of antibiotics at this stage!

Another elderly chap came in likewise with a chesty cough. As he started removing his jacket and woolly jumper, I couldn't help but notice a sickening stench emanating from his body. Not trying to be judgemental, I proceeded to lift his shirt only to reveal a rancid length of greasy linen strapped to his chest. He quite calmly stated that before considering bothering the doctor, he had tried his grandmother's home remedy for coughs; yes, goose fat, liberally applied to the skin. Like our 'Cupping man', topical goose fat is refuted to cure any number of skin conditions, help with diabetes and even cure piles. Even after years of medical training, I still cannot comprehend the vast range of differing cultural, religious and health beliefs that challenge us as doctors on a daily basis.

Within our practice population, we looked after a unit catering for quite severely mentally and physically handicapped individuals. The carers were always prepared to bring their patients to the surgery. I had one embarrassing encounter though when I called the next patient into my consulting room knowing they were from this specialist unit. In came a rather odd-looking guy being pushed in a wheelchair, his legs misshapen and deformed, by another chap. I looked up at the 'Helper' and asked what was wrong with his wheelchair-bound colleague.

To my utter surprise, the chap in the wheelchair piped out, "Doctor, he's the patient, I'm his care worker."

It didn't get any easier when shortly after this, another of the young residents of the unit came in, again in a wheelchair. I wasn't going to get caught out twice in one day. I promptly asked the 'Right' carer what the problem was and he replied that the young chap had not had his bowels open for several days. I decided that I'd need to examine his abdomen to make sure there was no sign of any obstruction. We manhandled him onto the clinical couch and loosened and lowered his jeans. I then made the biggest mistake of my life by pressing down on his abdomen. This was followed by the most ginormous evacuation of his bowels all over my couch. I immediately started to gag and was convinced that I was going to add to the variety of body fluids on the floor but managed to page one of my lovely nurses, Annie, who attended straight away and cleared everything up while I had to leave the room to breathe fresh air. Nurses, worth their weight in gold.

In the 16 years I worked as a GP in Essex, I consider that I had a pretty good working relationship with my patients, despite the fact that there was always a cluster of 'Heart sink' patients, those who seemed to always be attending the surgery and at worse always requesting a home visit, usually for unjustifiable reasons such as it was raining or that little Johnny was ensconced in his favourite TV programme.

I can only recall one occasion when a patient swore at me (At least face to face). We had recently moved into a custom-built medical centre with flash new computers and intercoms. I called my next patient in via the intercom. She sat down and I did my usual intro of asking how I could help her. I can't recall exactly what happened next but I think it was something to do with her demanding some particular medication. We had a heated debate culminating in her calling me a "F***ing useless doctor". After a few more expletives, she stamped out of the room slamming the door. I must admit that I was quite shaken by this experience. At that moment, someone knocked on my door. In came one of our medical receptionists.

"Peter," she said, "perhaps you should turn off your intercom. Your last consultation was just played over the whole building."

Still recovering, I paged my next patient to come in (Ensuring that everything was switched off this time). In came a lovely old lady, sat down and grinned. "I won't swear at you, Doctor," she said.

As GPs, we never really expected to be praised by our patients but sometimes it would have been welcome. During one very busy morning surgery, a middle-aged chap walked in saying that he had been getting some dull chest pains for a few days. Being overweight, a known smoker and with borderline high blood pressure, I didn't want to take any chances so got one of the practice nurses to do an ECG on him. To my horror, there were the tell-tail electrical signs of a heart attack. He looked remarkably well-considered but I did suggest that we get him admitted for further tests.

"OK, Doc, I'll just drive up to the hospital then," he calmly stated.

"I'd rather call for an ambulance to be on the safe side." I replied.

I duly settled him in one of the nurse's treatment rooms under supervision until I heard the ambulance siren fast approaching the surgery. The ambulance crew promptly got him onto a stretcher and wheeled him out to the waiting ambulance in our carpark. *Thank God,* I thought. Now he's in the hands of professionals. Seconds later, my phone rang. It was one of the receptionists requesting that I get to the ambulance ASAP. The back doors of the ambulance were still open. Why hadn't they set off? I could see immediately on the ECG that my patient had gone into Ventricular Fibrillation, a shockable heart rhythm but often fatal. Instinctively, we attached the defibrillator and shocked him. No response. We did it again and it was only after about six attempts, did his heart return to a viable stable rhythm and he regained consciousness. That was the rest of my day ruined and I spent hours pondering on what his outcome would be. Low and behold, about two weeks later, he returned to see me at the surgery. I was expecting a nice bottle of wine, box of chocolates or even a firm handshake showering me with gratitude and thanks for saving his life. No, not at all. He merely told me that he had only been given a two-week supply of heart medication by the hospital and wanted a repeat supply. Then he left.

Another patient from whom I thought I'd get some praise was a rather blunt but well-presented 50+ year old lady. She had seen all my partners over the proceeding 2-3 weeks with a persistent irritation on her scalp and neck. They had prescribed her a number of lotions and potions on the assumption that it was a form of eczema or psoriasis. None had worked. Being a conscientious doctor, I thought I'd best have a quick look at her scalp. To my horror as I parted her hair, a couple of fleas hopped out onto my desk. I quickly grabbed a length of sticky tape from a drawer and cornered them with it the first time. Holding the trapped fleas, I held up the tape to my startled patient expecting thanks for finally resolving her problem. But oh no. She merely accused me of planting them on her and stormed off in a huff (Yes, like we all keep a stash of fleas for such occasions).

During my 16 years in the practice, thankfully, I never had to attend a suicide although on one occasion a middle-aged chap came into my surgery with his wife feeling quite depressed because he had recently been made redundant. We had a chat and as he left, he turned and said that he'd get things sorted. I carried on with my surgery then about an hour later one of my partners knocked on the door and came in. As duty doctor, he had had a call from the same chap's wife saying that she could hear groaning from the bathroom but that the door was locked. She was worried that he might have had a heart attack. My partner forced the door open only to find the chap dead on the floor with a 6-inch carving knife through his heart.

There was one desperate young man who made at least three attempts to hang himself and somehow each time, I was the duty doctor called out. Not only that but on each occasion, the very same ambulance crew and local police attended. The poor chap obviously wasn't that determined to kill himself since on each occasion, he called his estranged girlfriend just before he jumped off the landing with a noose around his neck. His other mistake was that each time he used a dressing gown cord which naturally just stretched. I never ever found out what became of him.

When I first joined the practice, one of the partners was a member of BASICS, the British Association for Immediate Care. This meant that he could be called out to any accident or incident locally where there might be a delay in getting the emergency services on the scene. He loved it that he could attach a little green flashing strobe light onto the roof of his car just like Telly Savalas in Kojak and zoom off mid-surgery (Which didn't help the rest of us work wise). Anyway, I decided that I should also get a flashing green light for those 'Emergency' call outs. This was all very well until one night at about 2 am when I had a call to attend a chap with chest pain. I lived about 4–5 miles from where the patient was, so set off with flashing green strobes floodlighting the lanes. As I approached the village doing at least 50mph in a 30, I didn't spot the two police patrol cars stationed at the junction with officers in high viz jackets flagging me down. It must have looked surreal for the police to see a little white Fiat Panda 4x4 with a green flashing light on the roof. It did look a bit like a Sooty car. I wound my window down, shouted that I was a doctor attending a medical emergency and put my foot down. They never did follow it up.

Despite many colleagues mocking my little Fiat, it proved its worth the day after the October 1987 storm which created havoc on the roads around where we lived. My small 4x4 managed to get me into the surgery when most of the other staff were stranded at home. 1990 was my Annus Horribilis. I had had a nasty squash racket injury to my left eye resulting in an internal haemorrhage and temporary blindness resulting in a whole week of strict bed rest in hospital followed by another week at home recovering. Ironically and embarrassingly at the time, I was playing a chap much older than me but was obviously in the wrong position at the wrong time. Thankfully, the squash court was part of the officer's mess in Colchester Army Garrison and there just happened to be a consultant ophthalmologist and a general surgeon attending a formal dinner in the adjoining building. They attended to me immediately and I was then driven straight to the eye unit by my black tie dressed escorts. This, thankfully, eventually recovered then shortly after getting back to normal, my mother-in-law died after a car accident on her way to pick up our son from school. To cap it all, just before Christmas, my wife and I separated.

As an NHS GP, I inherited a number of longstanding patients, some of whom I looked after for 10–15 years. I'm sure patients gravitate to GPs they feel more comfortable with. In our practice at this time, although patients were registered with a particular GP, the patient was fully able to see whichever doctor they chose. Some would just see Dr X for their gynae problems and Dr Z for a rash etc.

One such lady was a frequent attendee at the surgery, often with quite vague symptoms which none of the partners could ever fathom out even when thoroughly investigated. She became what is often regarded as a 'Heart sink' patient. However, she and I developed quite a good working relationship and after multiple consultations, she said that she wanted to tell me something she had never disclosed to anyone, not even to her husband of many years. Then, she recounted how she was living in Singapore when the country was invaded by the Japanese in 1942. She described in sordid detail how she was gang-raped by a number of Japanese soldiers when she could have only been in her teens. At the time of her disclosure to me in the mid-1990s, she must have been in her 70s. To carry these horrid memories alone for so many years because she was too embarrassed to tell anyone had almost certainly had a prolonged detrimental effect on her health, physically and mentally. I provided her with some information about counselling available and strangely, she hardly re-attended the surgery again.

I only hope that our close doctor-patient relationship helped her to reconcile some of her awful wounds and that the remainder of her life was a little more bearable.

When I look back at my time at medical school and postgraduate training, over ten years in total, there was very little discussion about the psychology of illness. We were very much taught the established traditional 'Medical Model' in as much as symptoms=signs=diagnosis=treatment. Problem sorted.

It was only after studying two years for an MSc in general practice in the early 90s that we started taking into account things like the 'Patient's health beliefs' and asking our patients what they thought was causing their symptoms. Certainly in my NHS practice, as the new boy, some patients thought it very strange that I, the doctor, should ask for their opinion. The usual response was something like, "Well, you're the doctor, you tell me."

Whereas years ago, people with ailments would ask their neighbour or member of the family first what they thought about their symptoms, nowadays, sad to say, it's a quick Google search and rush to the doctor with the 100 possible causes of a headache!

And now of course, we have 'Zoom' and virtual consultations. I just hope that we do not lose the whole concept of general practice as being an art and a science.

# 1999–2000: Western Australia

Our pilot manoeuvred the Cessna 310 aircraft to the end of the unmade dusty landing strip. After a busy day in the clinic, we had packed up our kit and boarded the plane for the long flight back to our base. I contemplated how lucky I was to get the chance to work as a flying doctor in such an unusual and amazing place.

I, with a nurse and a student nurse, had flown out that morning to Balgo from Derby District Hospital, the regional hospital for the North West of Western Australia, and home of the Western Operations Royal Flying Doctor Service (RFDS). Balgo is one of Australia's most remote Aboriginal communities, located in the South Eastern Kimberley region of Western Australia on the northern edge of the Great Sandy Desert. It is some 600 km from Derby, nearly three hours flight each way, crossing nothing but scorched red earth.

Balgo had a population of 500–600. Although the settlement was served by a permanent resident nurse practitioner, a doctor only visited this community once a week, so one never knew quite what would present in the makeshift clinic. I was privileged to have this role for several months.

I often wondered how many of my GP contemporaries back in the UK would ever get to see elderly Aboriginals with the lifelong scarring and deformities from Leprosy, deal with venomous snakebites, hear some of the mystical 'Dreamtime' culture and history of these people or get the chance to do a combined consultation with a traditional Aboriginal Faith Healer?

As the plane accelerated along the rough terrain, a cloud of red dust filled the air. Then, up ahead we saw a small group of women hastily walking out onto the airstrip right in front of the aircraft, waving their arms frantically.

The pilot managed to come to a standstill just in front of the crowd.

We were then confronted by a young Aboriginal woman carrying a small bundle in her arms. It was a baby girl. We were told by the other women that her six months old daughter had been unwell with diarrhoea and vomiting for several days and that Mum had spent two days walking through the desert to get to the clinic in Balgo. At this point, the infant was unrousable, floppy and extremely dehydrated, just like a rag doll. We carried the infant back into the clinic. She desperately needed rehydrating. There were no veins visible. We tried to introduce a nasogastric tube into her stomach but there wasn't one fine enough to use.

Had we had a larger aircraft we could have taken the child and her mother with us back to base. As it was, there were already four of us and all our kit, hence no spare room. There was certainly nowhere anyone could have bedded down here for the night to wait for another plane the next day. In desperation, I called a senior doctor back in Derby hospital requesting that they send a flying doctor team. I was informed that this would take several hours. He advised me to try and perform an intraosseous transfusion to administer some fluids. I'd heard of such things but never seen one performed let alone do one myself. It involved screwing a corkscrew-like cannula into the bone marrow cavity in order to infuse some fluids (Electric-assisted devices are now the norm). The upper inner tibia is one of the preferred sites and as she was so small, we thought that this would be the best possible option. There was the constant fear of drilling right through the tibia, even splitting the bone or injuring surrounding soft tissues. The sad-looking child remained lifeless throughout, oblivious to the painful procedure being undertaken. After what seemed like a lifetime, we felt a 'Give' as the cannula slipped into the bone marrow cavity.

We attached a bag of fluids and to our amazement about 250 ml was infused in effortlessly. It was an amazing sight. Even as a doctor, I now still can't get over the thought of how fluid could be absorbed from the bone marrow cavity into the general circulation so easily.

It was a relief when we heard the flying doctor plane landing. As I handed over the infant to the flight nurse, she opened her eyes and whimpered. I was complimented for my medical skills by the experienced RFDS doctor who attended. I dared not tell him that it was a first for me!

I certainly needed a couple of ice-cold 'Tinnies' when I eventually got home that evening. What a day! But there would be a lot more exciting times ahead.

My baby made a full recovery and was soon reunited with her family.

I'd always had an inkling to work abroad but my first wife was never keen, so it didn't happen. Following the divorce, I then had an ideal opportunity to finally fulfil my ambition. My ex subsequently remarried so at least my two children would have a fatherly figure in the house if I was to be away for some considerable time. Thankfully, they all supported my desire to work abroad as long as the kids would get the opportunity to come out to visit me. I decided to leave my practice in 1998 after 16 years. At that time, I felt very guilty about leaving my partners and all the patients but I shouldn't have worried as when I finally returned to the UK after two years, most of my ex-patients hadn't even realised that I'd even been away. I saw an advert in one of the medical journals recruiting locum doctors to work in some of the rural parts of Western Australia. The agency was associated with the University of Western Australia in Perth which I felt gave it valid authenticity. I sent off my CV and a short while later, received an invitation to meet up with some Australian doctors in London for an interview. This proved successful and by the start of 1999, I was ready to go.

At this time, as I'd been a GP for so many years, I felt that I needed to brush up on some A&E type practice before flying out so I arranged to spend two weeks at a local hospital in Essex learning how to intubate and anaesthetise patients, interpret different X-rays, reduce and fix fractures and deal with a variety of medical emergencies, all of which would prove invaluable over the coming months.

The whole package seemed very reasonable. The locum agency would pay for my return flights, to and from Australia, provide a house and car and guarantee me full employment throughout my time there. On arrival in Perth, I was put up in a lovely apartment right in the city and for the first week, I spent the time with local GPs learning the way they worked.

My first assignment was for a month as a single-handed GP in a lovely coastal town called Kalbarri nestled inside a large national park about 600 km north of Perth. The practice there also had a small hospital complex with basic X-rays and blood testing facilities and run by very experienced nurses. I had flown up to Geraldton a couple of days beforehand to meet Betty who was the coordinator for the locum doctors in WA. Here, I had the use of a nice Toyota 4x4 and a beachside house for use as a bolt hole for when I was in between postings. Then on a Sunday afternoon, I drove the 150 km up to Kalbarri. I introduced myself to the hospital staff and then settled into my nice house overlooking the sea. It was early January, so the weather here was lovely. Early Monday morning I strode across to my new surgery and spent a very pleasant day seeing perhaps 10–15 patients with pretty much similar medical problems as I had been used to seeing in the UK. There would be however some unusual injuries in store ahead from snake bites, stonefish barbs, jellyfish reactions, embedded fishhooks and even stingray barb lacerations since this was a popular area for sea sports and fishing. At about 4 pm, thinking my day was done, I returned to my accommodation to contemplate my supper. Just before 8pm, I received a call from the duty nurses in the hospital saying that an elderly lady had just been admitted from a tourist coach passing through the area. By the time I arrived, they had already done an ECG which confirmed that she'd had a heart attack. We gave her oxygen and painkillers. *My job done,* I thought. I enquired to my efficient nurses what were we going to do with this lady.

"We need to get her to Perth," was the answer (All 600 km of it).

"So, does that mean contacting the flying doctors to come and collect her?"

How exciting I thought and only my first day. The next hitch was the fact that aircraft couldn't fly into Kalbarri at night as there were no landing lights, so we arranged to meet the aircraft in Northampton which was about 100 km inland through the park. This journey alone seemed to take forever due to the numerous kangaroos all over the road standing motionless and unperturbed by any oncoming traffic, hindering our speed. We finally reached the town's grass airstrip, by which time, the local volunteer fire service were erecting paraffin lamps along the airstrip. I looked like something out of an old film. We waited and waited until eventually, we heard the drone of a propeller aircraft overhead.

"That's them," said one of the nurses. 5–10 minutes passed and then the engine noise silenced. We phoned the flying doctor's HQ on the ambulance radio to find out what had happened to our plane. Apparently, because there was quite a harsh wind and the fact that the pilot would have to try and land on the grass by naked flames, he deemed it too unsafe. We were informed to travel further south (Another 50+km) to Geraldton airport (Not that far from where I had departed just the previous day) where at least there was a proper airstrip. We sped down the National Route 1 highway (Even though it was barely the width of one of our A roads) and eventually reached the airport and thankfully, the flying doctor plane was already there. The emergency doctor and nurse took over our patient and we watched as she was whisked off on her way to Perth. It was a long journey driving back to Kalbarri that night. There seemed to be even more kangaroos on the roads than earlier. I got home at 8am so my first day working in Australia had culminated in 12 hours just dealing with one patient. My first patient was due in at 08:30 that day so no time to recover. The only consolation was the fact that a week later we received a message from the doctors in Perth to say that my lady had made a full recovery.

The rest of my first month remained interesting and enjoyable and I think that the locals appreciated having UK doctors working there in these relatively remote areas. Despite being the only doctor in Kalbarri at this time and on-call 24/7, I still managed to get out and do quite a bit of snorkelling, sailing and horse riding but all had to be within calling distance in case of any emergencies.

For the next 20 or so months, I moved around the state spending between a week and several months at each location. Many were single-handed practices and getting a foreign GP locum was sometimes the only way that a resident doctor could get a break. It was impossible to drive to all the locations due to the vast distances involved. For example, the furthest north I worked was in a small dusty town called Halls Creek which was near the border of the northern territory some 2,800 km from Perth.

Considering that the state of Western Australia is about the same size as the whole of Western Europe, it has a population of less than three million, two-third of whom live in and around Perth. There is a substantial Aboriginal population in WA. Most lived in small townships constructed by the government and most had a resident schoolteacher, nurse practitioner and a chaplain. They were still basically nomadic and, on many occasions, when they had been helped by government agencies to irrigate the land and grow crops, they would pack up and go 'Walkabouts' for weeks on end. Perhaps they should not have been expected to adapt or conform completely to westernised ideas and values.

One of my roles at several of the practices was to be flown out to various remote townships, some of them 2-3 hours into the desert and conduct as good a general practice service as facilities would allow. I have to say that during my time in WA, I undertook more medical/surgical procedures than in all the years before.

In one of the coastal practices, I was the sole doctor. A farmer was brought in who had fallen off his quad bike rounding up his sheep, sustaining a chest injury. He was having difficulties breathing and a subsequent CXR revealed that he had a haemo-pneumothorax (A damaged collapsing lung). We were a long way from any major hospital, and despite radioing the flying doctors, was told that there were no planes available until the following day. I managed to call a consultant chest physician in Perth for advice.

"You need to insert a chest drain," he instructed.

One small problem though. I had never inserted a chest drain.

"It's easy," he replied and directed me to an intriguing DIY surgery book which was in the coffee room for this sort of everyday procedure. I scanned the relevant chapter on chest drains; where to make the cut, which rib space and how to connect up all the drainage/suction apparatus (To help re-inflate the lung). I confidently advised the patient that he needed this surgical procedure and successfully achieved a good result. I didn't have the heart to reveal that this was the first such procedure I had performed. Thankfully, he made a good recovery.

Feeling that I was a wasted chest physician after the above, about a week later, an elderly lady was brought in from a passing coach trip through WA. She was extremely breathless and distressed. A CXR showed that the whole of one lung was a 'White out', a term used when the lung pleural space is completely filled with fluid usually from a sinister cause. I did try the flying doctor tactic again as I knew she needed to have the fluid taken off her chest but once more I was told that they could not get a plane up to us until the following day, by which time it might be too late to save her. Once again, I called the chest unit in Perth for advice.

"Just stick a wide bore needle between the ribs nearest the densest area of fluid," came the response.

*Here we go again,* I thought. I had done similar minor procedures like this in the UK but that was in a busy well-staffed hospital with plenty of potential backup if anything went wrong. Sitting the old lady up on the medical couch, I put some local anaesthetic at the site to make the stab. In went the large needle and straight away a milky fluid started pouring out. We attached a drainage tube to a bottle. Within about 30 minutes, some 1500 ml had drained and not understandably, she felt 100% better. We kept a close eye on her overnight on the ward and thankfully, a flying doctor plane arrived the following morning to take her down to Perth. I later found out that the fluid around her lung was due to an underlying lung cancer but unfortunately, never found out how she faired.

I had a very pleasant locum job in a small coastal town called Exmouth. One day a week, I was flown across a large bay to do an outreach Aboriginal clinic in a commune called Onslow. By road, it was over 400 km and would have taken over four hours each way as it was a very tortuous coastline. From the air, one could regularly see pods of whales within the bay. This area of WA is also famous for the Ningaloo Reef, a huge coral reef that many have said is a rival to the Great Barrier Reef. It was here that I learnt to scuba dive. The highlight of my time here however was the chance to go out on a whale shark encounter. We went out on a small powerboat whilst a spotter plane scoured the sea from above. Then the call came in that they had spotted several just ahead of us. We donned our masks and flippers and jumped off the back of the boat. Once the bubbles had dispersed, we looked up and there swimming along the side of the boat were several huge whale sharks, estimated to be about 8–10 metres long. They moved so slowly that for a while one could swim right alongside them as they were only a few feet under the surface. One could easily have touched them as they were so docile but this was discouraged. In all, we saw about six of them that day. Luckily, I had purchased a cheap disposable underwater camera and despite having little time to compose and plan any photos, I managed to get some amazing closeup pictures of these incredible creatures. It was one of the most memorable days I'd ever had.

I worked several times in a private GP practice in Geraldton. Most patients were covered by the medicare system but practices could charge over and above what the health insurance would reimburse. The GPs also had admitting rights to the local hospital and took it in turns to work in the A&E department there which made the job quite variable. On one particular morning, a middle-aged woman came in with abdominal pains. I suspected that she might have a gallbladder problem. I arranged for her to have an ultrasound scan at the private clinic in town which they did 30 minutes later. Shortly after that, I received a phone call confirming that she had gallstones and an inflamed gallbladder. I referred her to a surgeon who saw her at 2 pm and by 5 pm, she had had her gallbladder removed! And all covered by her health insurance. I sometimes think that we in the UK could learn some lessons from how other countries organise their health services.

Whilst working in a small GP led hospital in Carnarvon (about 900 km north of Perth) I was the duty doctor one evening when I received a radio message to say that a fisherman on a lobster trawler had caught one of his hands in the metal cables used to drag up the pots. They were still quite a way out to sea at this time but he gave me an ETA of 4–5 hours later which meant he would arrive at the hospital about 3 am. So much for my beauty sleep. He duly arrived and asked me to patch up his hand as he didn't want to miss the next tide out back on his trawler. To him, time was money. To my horror, on removing some very blood-stained grubby bandages, he had traumatically amputated two fingers. There was little soft tissue remaining, just bony stumps. "This is a plastic surgery job," I told him. But the nearest unit would be Perth and would need a plane. In my short time here so far, I didn't have much faith in this organisation which on the TV always responded to any need anywhere, anytime. The chap asked me to patch him up. I'd never done anything like this before but using common sense, good wound debridement, cleaning and a bit of bone nibbling, I managed to get enough skin to cover the open wounds.

He finally lifted up his rather deficient hand and declared, "Not a bad job, mate." He was back on his trawler a couple of hours later.

I'd always enjoyed minor surgery and stitching up little cuts and lacerations. My surgical skills were however fully tested when another burly farmer came into the clinic one day with his upper leg all bandaged up. He had had a fall from his motorcycle and ripped open his thigh from the handlebars. What a mess it looked; a flap of skin hanging off bigger than my outstretched hand. I could see all the muscles beneath the gap. I suggested that we should transfer him to a hospital as it was going to need quite a bit of sowing up. We were only about two hours from Perth on this occasion but he insisted that I should do the deed. After 80 individual stitches, I had managed to close the huge void and it looked pretty neat. He left happy and came back about ten days later to have all the stitches removed. It looked amazingly good I have to say.

Whilst working at the same practice, another farmer came in one day and asked if I'd like to go up in a glider the following weekend. I'd never done so before so jumped at the chance. What I hadn't realised is that he would be my pilot. He flew Lancaster bombers in WW2 so must have been in his 90s. The take-off was pretty scary as they used an old farm truck to pull the glider along a very uneven field. It bounced up and down so much that I was convinced that we were going to plough into a ditch or hedge. Once high enough, he released the pull tie. Hopefully, it wouldn't jam, or we'd be pulled back to earth with a vengeance. It was only then that I had the horrific thought of what do I do if he pegs it whilst we're stuck up in the clouds. I didn't enjoy the experience and don't ever intend to go up in one again.

I'm normally quite a good flyer but there's a huge difference between a Boeing 747 and a four-seater Piper single prop aircraft. I certainly did my fair share of flying in the latter during my time in WA. The weather in WA could be quite varied and seasonal. I got very used to sudden drops in altitude due to adverse updrafts and turbulence. Willy willies, derived from the Aboriginal language, otherwise known as dust devils or tornados were very common during the tropical seasons and quite dramatic when seen from above. On one particular flight from one of the desert settlements, there was just me and the young pilot. Up ahead there were signs of a huge storm with black clouds, thunder and lightning. He indicated that he would have to fly up above it to avoid the weather as it was too wide across to go around. As we ascended above 10,000 feet, I saw him rummaging around on the floor then a few moments later, he produced an oxygen mask and gas bottle. "Where's my oxygen?" I enquired.

"You don't get any. It's only necessary for the pilot to use oxygen above 10,000 feet." I was so glad when we had passed the storm.

In Derby, a small town in the north of WA, I worked in a GP led district hospital. There were six GPs including myself, the others all Australian. GPs here often had additional specialist training such as anaesthetics, obstetrics and general surgery. Somehow, I got pinged for paediatrics which meant attending all deliveries just in case of any problems. As it happened, Aboriginal women were usually very natural deliverers. Luckily, I had done a six-month paeds job during training but was a long time before and I was certainly a bit rusty. About once a month, a visiting surgeon and gynaecologist would come for a week at a time and do whatever procedures that were deemed routine and didn't require transfer all that way down to Perth. Also, the traditional Aboriginals often had a bit of distrust of westernised medicine and preferred to be treated locally.

Derby was the regional royal flying doctor service hub with a couple of Beechcraft King Air turboprop aircraft and fully trained flight nurses. Initially, when I started there, the GPs at the hospital acted as the flight doctors. No, we didn't fly the planes ourselves (As most people think when you mention this role). Each aircraft had two pilots. We could be called out to any medical incident such as a heart attack, car crash, just anything. In addition to this, the GPs had allocated Aboriginal townships to visit, usually once a week. Some were drivable but most were by aircraft, well into the Red Desert.

I worked in several different Aboriginal outreach clinics. The townships themselves had been constructed by the government so that families had their own property with proper kitchens and bathrooms. However historically, Aboriginals had not lived in houses as many were nomadic. Within a few months of occupancy, most of the houses had had their windows and doors torn down to fuel the outdoor fires. Most of them slept outside, just a bare mattress on the soil. I won't describe the state of the bathrooms. I was shown inside one house and was horrified to see a whole dead cow suspended from a ceiling raft in the middle of the living area. The flies were something else. In some communities, there was a small store that sold food and other necessities but this only really encouraged them to eat unhealthy processed food. Obesity was rife. The incidence of diabetes, kidney failures and heart disease was astonishing. Seeing a 25-year-old Aboriginal woman die of a heart attack was so sad. Most townships had a basic school and a first aid building run by nurses who lived within the communities for up to six months at a time. I found a day working in such environments quite taxing.

One of the main problems having white Caucasian doctors and nurses to treat the Aboriginal people was the significant differences in cultural beliefs especially when it came to treating various illnesses. A prime example was the treatment of skin infections which was rife. Normally, I would prescribe an antibiotic 3-4 times a day for 1-2 weeks. Most Aboriginals either swallowed the whole lot in one go or took a couple of doses then bin the rest. Many were illiterate so it was no point writing instructions on a prescription. Instead, we'd often use stick-on pictorial labels depicting sunrise, midday and sunset which indicated when they should take their tablets. Another way around this was for us to give them a 4ml intramuscular injection of Penicillin (Not a pleasant feeling for anyone) whilst we had them in the clinic. How much this helped it was difficult to judge.

I had my first experience with an Aboriginal witch doctor/faith healer in one of the desert townships. I was running my normal weekly clinic seeing a young lad who just felt unwell. I examined him but couldn't find anything amiss. Out of nowhere came this elder whom I was told was a faith healer who started chanting and waving his hands all over my patient. Both of them looked like they were in a trance. After about 15 minutes, the healer told me via one of the nurse assistants to check the boy's kidneys as he felt that that was the cause of his illness. I felt I had to play along so I got him to produce a urine sample and dip stuck it which to my complete surprise and horror, showed blood and masses of white cells confirmed that he did indeed have a kidney/renal tract infection. We flew him off to our hospital in Derby where tests confirmed that he had a severe kidney infection which could have caused sepsis even death had he not been treated. Unfortunately, I never got the chance to meet up with my faith healer colleague again but the experience did instil in me how we as doctors should not dispel other health beliefs and practices handed down through the ages.

Most of the isolated farmsteads in WA were provided with emergency medical chests with a detailed list of all the drugs and medical equipment therein. It was common practice for patients to radio into the hospital or flying doctor centre depending on the location where appropriate advice could be given. This way, individuals could be prescribed drugs such as antibiotics and painkillers without the long trudge (If at all possible) to see a doctor. Also, many of the dirt track roads became completely impassable during the tropical rainy season.

All over WA but particularly in the Derby area, I was quite puzzled about the number of Aboriginals who had quite bad skin lesions often looking like chronic non-healing ulcers in addition to those with missing fingers and toes and even parts of their nose. It became obvious when I was seeing one of these individuals in the clinic and one of the nurses said to me, "How much Leprosy have you seen?" To me, Leprosy was a disease of the Middle Ages but not so. A Leprosarium was established in Derby in 1936 and didn't close until 1986, the very last of its kind in Australia, when treatment with a combination of anti-bacterial drugs was discovered that could treat it, although patients often had to take these for 6–12 months. Unfortunately, the residual scarring and deformities lasted for life. It is estimated that over 1000 patients with Leprosy passed through the Derby Leprosarium. In the adjoining graveyard, there are nearly 400 buried.

On the subject of skin conditions, I've always prided myself as being quite good at spot-diagnosing an array of skin lesions, rashes etc. However, I was caught out by a young lad who came in complaining about a red itchy rash but only over his face and genitals. I racked my brains to come up with a logical diagnosis but this one had me completely stumped. I managed to collar one of my Australian doctor colleagues. I explained the rash and asked what he thought. The first thing he said was, "What job does he do?"

I went back to the patient and asked.

"I'm a mango fruit picker," he replied.

I was none the wiser but on informing my colleague, he merely said, "That'll be it then. We see it all the time with mango pickers but just advise him to wash his hands before and after a wee and not to wipe his face after either." Apparently, mangos have an irritant compound within the peel similar to that found in poison ivy. It certainly put me off eating mangoes. Ironically, a few weeks after the baby incident, I was back at the same Aboriginal township doing a clinic. Again, we had just finished for the day and were all loaded up ready to fly back to base. As we departed from the clinic, a small group of women arrived at the entrance. A middle-aged lady appeared, clutching her blood-covered arm. Pulling back the dressings, I couldn't believe that she had a pair of metal garden secateurs embedded through her forearm. Fearing that she might have damaged some major arteries or nerves, I resisted removing the weapon as if she started haemorrhaging, we would be stuffed. It appears that a routine domestic dispute with her husband had triggered off this rather gruesome act. On this occasion, we managed to take her back to the hospital on our plane. Luckily, we had a visiting surgeon there at that time. X-rays revealed that the secateurs had completely cut through both radius and ulna bones. On surgical exploration, thankfully, there was no blood vessel or nerve damage. This was another first for me, inserting metal plates to secure her two fractures (At least with some supervision this time).

The same surgeon was always very keen to teach fellow doctors and even during my relatively short time working in Derby, he had me performing appendicectomies and other quite difficult orthopaedic procedures.

After a number of flights into the Red Desert with the same pilot, Matt, I started to get a bit apprehensive as to what I would do if anything happened to him whilst we were mid-air. On quite a lot of these flights, there was just him and me. The Aboriginal settlement of Balgo, my allotted community in the Kimberley region of WA, was about 600km (400 miles) from our base in Derby. Most of the time one could only see limitless desert up to the horizon as there were few natural landmarks to identify or guide us, certainly no towns, roads or rivers in this huge region. As a result of all this, I had some very basic flying instruction from him, learning how to alter the speed, fuel mix and steering of the plane, and how one could engage and disengage the auto-pilot.

Now feeling a little more confident, I felt that I could relax a bit more during these long fights.

A week or two later, I was the duty doctor in Derby A&E when a call came through urgently requesting a doctor to attend the nearby dental clinic which was just behind the main hospital. On entering, I was informed that a patient had collapsed unconscious whilst having a local dental anaesthetic.

To my horror, it was my faithful young pilot, Matt. Luckily, he roused after a few minutes on oxygen. It was uncertain whether the dental surgeon had accidentally injected the local anaesthetic into a blood vessel but in view of the uncertainty as to whether it was due to this or perhaps some other possible cardiovascular mishap, the poor chap was naturally grounded from further flying. He had spent the previous two years accumulating a respectable number of flying hours in small prop aircraft in the hope of one day being able to apply as a commercial pilot, and being an Aussie, naturally wanted to join Quantas. Alas, this was now all ruined. By the time that I left this job, his future and career aspirations remained in the balance.

I had just finished one of my weekly outreach clinics in Balgo and was getting ready to go out to the waiting aircraft. At that moment, one of the nurses came rushing in to say that the 'Mad woman of Balgo' had pitched up at the clinic and that she was extremely agitated and acting strange. Apparently, she had lived in the outback for a number of years and was rarely seen. So, why did she turn up just when I was there! I was taken into an adjoining room where this thin dishevelled lady wearing rags was crawling around the floor talking incoherently.

She had matted hair, rotten teeth and smudged makeup on her face. She then started trying to pull on my clothes and undo my shoelaces. When I tried to approach her, she crawled and cowered under a desk sobbing. At this point in the day, I was just keen to get back to base. This was the last thing I needed. I made an executive decision to try and sedate her so that we could assess her better. I asked the nurse to draw me up a syringe of Haloperidol, an anti-psychotic drug.

At that very moment, the 'Mad woman of Balgo' stood up, removed her wig and false teeth laughing. It was none other than the flight nurse who'd I'd flown out with earlier in the day. "We do that little trick to all the new doctors," she said. The rest of the staff found the whole thing highly amusing but they'd probably seen it many times before. She was so close to getting a large needle of Haloperidol into her backside! She did prove to be a great asset to me as the 'Newbie' with her long track record and expertise as an Aussie flight nurse.

After regularly visiting various Aboriginal settlements, I got a bit of a following, I suppose because they didn't even see many white people for months at a time. On one occasion, an elder came into the clinic clutching a rolled-up canvass under his arm. I tried to engage with him but was then told by my nurse that he couldn't talk because he had no tongue. It appears that he had a bit of a disagreement with some other Aboriginal men when he was a young man and as a result had his tongue chopped off. Anyway, I was informed that he was a traditional painter and was keen to know if I wanted to purchase this painting. He unrolled it and held it up. To me, it epitomised Aboriginal life and culture. I indicated to the old man that I would be interested in buying the painting. But how much? After all, there couldn't be much demand for such artwork in the middle of the WA desert. It was three hours by plane to the nearest town and there were no constructed roads anywhere nearby. He raised his hand holding out his five fingers. It can't just be five dollars I thought so I got $50 from my wallet and held it up. He looked a bit hesitant but grabbed the money and left abruptly. Later that day, I got back to the hospital and happened to meet up with a couple of the Australian doctors.

"Look what I bought from an Aboriginal guy today. I paid 50 dollars for it."

"Who was the artist?" one of them asked. I showed him the signature on the painting.

"Christ mate," he exclaimed. "He's a really well-known artist. He regularly exhibits in Perth and Sydney. His paintings often fetch 500 dollars."

For a couple of months, I did a weekly clinic at an Aboriginal community called Mowanjun, about 10 km from Derby. There was a small hut there displaying traditional Aboriginal artwork. On one occasion as I skimmed through the various paintings, I was struck by a print of some strange depiction of human figures, some almost looking alien in character. As I picked up the print, a voice behind me said, "That's a good choice. It's one of mine." At the bottom of the picture was written 'Gulingi Wandjinas (A reference to the Rain spirits) a limited edition print mark of 4/30 and his signature, Donny Woolagoodja.

We spent the next hour discussing Aboriginal art and its origins. Donny had been born in the Kunmunya Presbyterian Mission in remote NW Kimberley in 1947. His father was a renowned lawman and medicine man who some say was the last great man of power of the Wororra people. Donna was educated in two worlds, understanding the white world of the

Mission whilst deeply upholding the traditional beliefs of his people. He became one of the foremost artists of Mowanjun and in fact, the 12-metre giant Namarali Wandjina painting featured in the opening ceremony of the Sydney 2000 Olympic Games was his work.

Wandjina style is a type of depiction in Australian cave painting of figures that represent mythological beings associated with the creation of the world. They are only found in the Kimberley region of NW Australia and only a few artists ever win the right to depict Wandjinas as they are regarded as being so sacred.

Wandjina figures are depicted without mouths and the enlarged faces are always painted white. The head is usually surrounded by a red halo or horseshoe motif with lines radiating outward (Which certainly reminds one of alien beings). Wandjina figures have a predominantly white and ochre colouration because they symbolise the essence of water and blood.

I came to realise that 'Dreamtime' is a commonly used term for describing important features of Aboriginal spiritual beliefs and existence. Aboriginals believe that Dreamtime was way back at the very beginning and that the land and the people were created by spirits.

Dreaming is as important to Aboriginal people as the Christian Bible and the whole ethos of Christian belief is to the devout Christian. The past of the spirit ancestors which live on in the legends are handed down through stories, art, ceremony and songs.

Now, every time I walk past one of the several Aboriginal artworks at home that I purchased in WA, I have very fond memories of those days treating and hopefully, making a small difference in their lives.

Domestic violence seemed quite a problem amongst the Aboriginal population. Police were few and far between in the remote areas of WA and it appeared that in a lot of cases they relied on local people to resolve local issues. I came across a lot of alcohol and drug-related problems throughout my time in WA. There appeared to be quite an association between acute mental illnesses and cannabis use. I was told by a local chap in Fitzroy Crossing in the very north of WA that an area of the township had so many beer cans piled up that it could be seen from outer space. Whether this was actually true, I never did find out. I was also particularly concerned about how many people were regularly taking opiate drugs for conditions such as 'Chronic low back pain'.

One such example was a middle-aged white lady who presented to A&E saying that she needed treatment for a migraine attack. She appeared very evasive and reluctant to engage. She had a large brimmed hat and sunglasses, I imagined because she was finding the light aggravating. After a cursory examination, for which she refused to remove her sunglasses, I offered her a standard migraine drug. She then told me that the only drug that helped her pain was Pethidine 100mg IM. It was only then that I noticed her pinpoint pupils which can be a sure sign of opiate misuse. I refused her demands at which point she hurriedly exited the hospital. I later found out from some of my other colleagues that she was a regular attendee in the area for the same rouse.

One day I was the duty doctor in the Derby hospital A&E department when an elderly Aboriginal lady was brought in covered in cuts and bruises. It transpired that her husband had beaten her up. We were of the opinion that we should report him to the local police. She assured us that this wouldn't be necessary. "We have ways of dealing with these things,'" she replied. Sure enough, about an hour later, an old boy was pushed into A&E on a stretcher also very battered and bruised. "There's my husband," said the old lady. It transpired that her family members had exacted suitable payback on her husband. To cap it all, about another hour later, we caught both of them sharing a bed in the sideward.

One of the most unpleasant duties I had to perform whilst working in Derby was to examine and obtain forensic samples from two alleged rape victims, both Aboriginal, one a five-year-old boy and the other an 80-year-old lady. I left this job shortly after so never did find out what the outcomes were but it was one of the more unpleasant aspects of the job I had to perform.

We never knew what would present to the A&E department. One day an old Aboriginal man came in for quite a minor problem. I couldn't help but notice a huge protuberant scar across his forehead. On closer inspection, it became obvious that it was a row of very embedded metal clips often used to close wounds. Usually, these are removed 7–10 days after insertion. How long had my chap had his in?

"About 18 months ago," he told me.

I merely told him that his wound had healed very well and he contently left.

Another elderly Aboriginal chap came into the clinic with some paperwork to be completed for his driving licence. This did seem quite odd given that there were few made-up roads around there. The last set of traffic lights I had seen was back in Perth nearly 2400 km south. He needed to have his vision recorded so I took him over to the eye chart hanging on the wall. "Cover one eye and tell me what letter is on the top line (A huge letter A)." There was complete silence. "Can you see any letters on the chart?" I asked.

"Nope," he responded.

*Christ,* I thought, *he's totally blind. I can't pass him fit to drive.*

At that moment, one of the regular nurses came past. I told her of my predicament but she just laughed and told me that Fred couldn't read or write. She then turned the eye chart around to reveal not letters but a series of animal pictures of varying sizes. "Right, Fred," she said to the old man, "what are these?" Without hesitation, he started rattling off ever-smaller and smaller images of animals- kangaroo, crocodile, parrot, emu, camel etc. That taught me a great lesson.

A more unusual A&E encounter occurred when a couple of young Aboriginal children came in clutching something in their hands. "What have we got here?" I asked.

"It's a baby Echidna," (Sometimes known as a spiny anteater) they replied. I was at this point none the wiser. The trouble was that this baby creature had tried to get into a beer can and become wedged halfway. With the help of one of the nurses, we got some metal cutters and freed the poor little thing and gave it back to the children.

"By the way," I asked, "what became of its mother?"

"Oh, we ate her."

Another five-year-old Aboriginal boy was brought in by his mother as he had been complaining of some buzzing in one of his ears for about a week. On examining him, I could see something blocking his ear canal. I cautiously used a pair of forceps to remove whatever the offending foreign object was. To my horror, it was a live cockroach.

One of the most disturbing things I experienced in WA was a ritual undertaken on adolescent Aboriginal boys, usually between 10 and 16 years of age to signify a rite of passage, often referred to as the Walkabout. They would be taken off into the outback and live with the male elders for weeks at a time to make the spiritual and traditional transition into manhood. The ritual itself then involved doing a radical circumcision and subincision of the urethra often along the whole length of the penis often only using a sharp flint or a rusty old razor blade. This was not an optional choice. In most cases, there was no form of anaesthetic, maybe some herbal hypnotic and often the boys were forcibly constrained spread-eagled on the floor during the procedure. This was usually associated with the incision of scars on their chest, shoulders, arms and buttocks. I recall seeing half a dozen adolescent lads waiting in one of the remote clinics who had all had this procedure done a day or two before. My Aussie nurse that day knew what they had been through but didn't pre-warn me of what I was about to witness. I felt physically sick. I think my facial expression revealed this when I hurried out of the clinic in disbelief. Their penises looked like they had been put through a mangle. A spatchcock chicken would describe the appearances graphically (Apologies for the analogy). Secondary infections were rife. The only haemostatic agent used during the operation was hot ash dusted over the affected parts post-surgery. All I could do for these lads was to offer advice on keeping the wounds clean and antibiotics as needed. I continually wondered how these men would ever pee normally again and also how they would inseminate their partners. No doubt the tradition continues to this day. I never did find out whether the young female Aboriginal girls endured a similar ordeal.

It was Christmas Day (1999) at the end of my first year in WA. We had an amazing day with an outdoor party by the pool with all the medical staff in some 35C heat. The BBQ was in action for the whole day and many a tinny of the cold stuff was had. On Boxing Day, I was not on duty and some of the local Aboriginals asked if I wanted to go out for some 'Bush tucker'. I had instructions to meet them at their camp. I had the use of a large Toyota Land cruiser jeep which was just as well as by the time we set off, I must have had 12-15 of them on board, some of the little ones even hanging on the roof racks. I had toddlers, mums and dads and several elder grannies. We drove for about an hour into the desert then finally stopped in a dried-up riverbed. Instantly, all the kids jumped out and ran off down the channel. I had no idea what they were doing. They started poking around in some burrows in the earth bare-handed, not something I would have done knowing what might be inside them. A while later, there was a great deal of screaming and singing then the appearance of all the children carrying a dead, four-feet long Goanna (Monitor lizard). This was triumphantly presented to the elders who by now had got a good fire going. I'm not sure now whether they gutted the beast but either way the huge creature was buried in a pile of ash and left to cook. I wish I hadn't been there when they removed the ash to reveal a very dark burnt crusty lizard, head and claws still attached. As I was the guest of honour, one old lady proceeded to rip off a leg and ceremoniously hand it to me. It looked like a piece of burnt fat and smelt disgusting. I pretended to nibble a bit of the rancid flesh then managed to dispose of it when I went back to the jeep to get the kids some sweets. Thinking this was it as far as my 'Bush tucker' initiation was concerned, I assumed that we would soon head back to the town. But oh no. Next were the honey ants. These were huge things, about 1.5 cm long. Quite a delicacy for the Aboriginals apparently. The knack here was to grab the ant just below its head and front legs then suck the 'Honey' out of its plump abdomen. I did it once but that was it. Sometimes they would drop whole nests of the things into a vat of hot water and make a delicious broth which I was told had some medicinal properties.

Thankfully, nobody produced a witchetty grub. That would have been the final straw. How the contestants of *I'm a celebrity, get me out of here* did it, I'll never know.

The last example of native delicacies involved the Aboriginals picking leaves off a small bush then grinding them up in a clay dish. Once in paste form, they threw small amounts into a small creek. Minutes later, a whole batch of stunned fish floated to the surface ready to be gathered for another gourmet treat.

Another exposure to 'Bush tucker' was when I was driving through the desert towards one of the settlements. I saw a couple of Aboriginal men in the river nearby. They obviously didn't get much through trade as they called for me to stop. They already had a wood fire burning on the riverbank. "Do you fancy some bush tucker mate?" one of them asked.

I enquired what they were going to cook.

"Kangaroo steaks," they replied. I had envisaged that they had spent the morning stroking a kangaroo, killing it with a spear then gutting and filleting it.

"Where did you get the kangaroo?" I asked.

"We got it from the freezer store in Woolworths," they replied. So much for my romantic image of this noble race. I thanked them for the offer but chose to drive on.

But…a couple of weeks later, I was invited around to have dinner with a couple of Aussie hospital staff. After a few beers and glasses of wine, we sat down to eat. "What have we got to eat?" I asked.

"An Australian classic, mate," was the response. "Kangaroo tail casserole."

I have to say that I've had much worse but have never eaten any since.

The only real bush tucker that I did enjoy was when a group of us went out fishing for freshwater shrimps and mud crabs using nets. I was warned by the more knowledgeable Aussies never to throw the net into the river from the same position twice. Why not? Because the crocodiles are clever enough to latch on to this and could easily jump up and take you out. Although the freshwater crocodiles tended only to be about four-feet long and relatively harmless, the larger saltwater crocs were often 15–18 feet long and a completely different matter, occasionally migrating quite far inland. I was aware of at least one aboriginal boy taken by one of these nearby whilst I was there.

Derby was surrounded by some spectacular scenery and an amazing coastline. It was great to walk through some of the vast gorges as long as one kept a watch out for the crocodiles. One weekend, I was on a walk with a work colleague, Delia, an Australian GP. We were about an hour up the gorge and chatting and I happened to say to Delia that in the year that I'd been in WA I hadn't seen a live snake (One saw a lot of dead ones on the roads). At that moment, Delia quietly said, "Don't move, Peter, there's a Western Brown snake on its haunches on the path about 18 inches ahead of you." I slowly turned to see this snake whose head was at the level of my groin. We froze for what seemed like a lifetime until the snake obviously got bored and slithered into the undergrowth.

"Would you have sucked the poison out if I'd been bitten?" I joked.

"No F***ing chance," she replied.

Derby was quite a small remote dusty town; a few basic shops, a couple of pubs, one hotel (Basic) and the regional hospital where I worked. For a decent meal or nice beach, one had to drive across the country to Broome on the western coast, some 200 km, about a two hours' drive. I planned to do this one weekend and have some lunch by the sea just to get away from my work environment. Just as I was leaving the hospital, one of the Aussie nurses asked if I would let her come for the ride as she didn't have her own transport. On arrival in Broome, I didn't feel that I could just dump her so offered to buy her lunch. We found a lovely beachside restaurant, sat down and started looking at the menu. She went off to the loo. A waiter came over and asked if I wanted any wine.

"Yes please," I said. "What Chardonnays have you got?"

"Would that be the red or white, sir?" he asked.

With some desperation, I replied, "Chardonnay is the classic white wine." Off he went.

A few minutes later, my nurse friend returned. "You'll never guess," I said, "I asked the waiter for a bottle of Chardonnay and he asked me whether I wanted red or white."

"Yeh right," she answered, "and which one did you choose?"

The wildlife in WA was amazing. I still remember seeing my first wild camels walking along the side of the main coastal road. Apparently, WA is now home to the largest herd of feral camels in the world. They were originally imported into Australia from British India and Afghanistan during the nineteenth century for transport and construction during the colonisation of the central and western parts of Australia. Many were released into the wild after motorised transport replaced the use of camels in the early twentieth century. It is estimated that the number of camels may now outnumber red kangaroos by 100 to one! Although it was uncommon to see camels on my travels, when one appreciates that WA is the size of Western Europe, it's not hard to see why they rarely ventured into the more populated areas of the state.

Emus were always a lovely sight especially when one saw 10–12 tiny chicks following a parent in a perfect line.

I experienced some of the wildlife wonders of the ocean in WA, especially around Shark Bay and Exmouth, about 1,250 km north of Perth. From the air, one could frequently see humpback, southern right and blue whales migrating along the coastline (Particularly when I flew across from Exmouth to Onslow to conduct outreach clinics).

I was lucky enough to see dugongs, dolphins and sharks at close quarters and even a chance to swim alongside several Whale sharks.

Freshwater crocodiles were very common along the many rivers and gorges. I did see a couple of huge 'Salties', extremely dangerous saltwater crocs, when in Derby.

Having been working in WA for 18 months, I decided to take some time off. My two children, James, aged 15, and Celine, aged 13, flew over from the UK as it was their summer holidays. British Airways staff were fantastic in supervising them on such a long flight via Singapore. I met them in Perth where we had a few days rest for them to recover from the jet lag. I wanted to show them as much of the country as I had seen so I hired a 4x4 Land Rover Cruiser and we spent the next four weeks driving up the WA coast, stopping somewhere different every few days. We got as far as Kununurra just up near to the northern territory border. The car logged up 4,000 miles in total. During this epic journey, we went scuba diving, horse riding, camel riding, canoeing, sailing, outback camping, hand feeding dolphins, and even a helicopter ride over the Bungle Bungles, a World Heritage site within the Kimberley region of WA.

To me, the highlight of our adventure was to drive through the Gibb River Road, a 400-mile dirt track from Derby in the west to Kununurra in the east. The road was only first constructed in the 1960s to transport cattle from outlying stations to the ports of Derby and Wyndham. A 4x4 vehicle was almost certainly a must given the number of rivers one had to negotiate. Much of the road itself was extremely uneven with large ditches and burrows (Locally known as corrugations). One could rarely drive faster than 20–30 mph. This was obviously not what another couple thought. Towards the end of our cross-country expedition, we were due to reach an isolated farmstead for an overnight stay. A few miles before this, we came across an overturned vehicle on the road and could see a chap kneeling over and attending to a blood-soaked woman. Had we not been on the road at that time heaven knows when another vehicle would have appeared? We rushed to the scene. It appears they were a French couple on their honeymoon. They had obviously been driving too fast on such a perilous road and just lost control. The girl had some quite nasty head and facial injuries. The guy was extremely shaken, one ear badly lacerated. My kids were amazing. Celine immediately found our first aid pack and started cleaning up the poor woman. James meanwhile helped collect some of their essential baggage and belongings from their trashed vehicle. Their vehicle would not be going anywhere so we bundled them both into our Cruiser and continued towards the farmhouse. What a relief to find the place as we didn't have a satnav. The farm station merely had a small old hand-painted wooden sign pointing up an even more unmade track. On arrival, I rushed in and got the owner and his staff to come out and help us move the casualties. I carried on attending to their wounds. I asked the owner to contact the flying doctors and get the couple airlifted out to the hospital. Kununurra was probably only about 100 km further up the Gibb River road but not a journey one would want to attempt in the dark. Why was I not surprised to hear that they could not get a plane out that late as it would be dark soon and there were no landing light facilities near the farm? They would send a plane out first thing the next day. What was I supposed to do with the two casualties overnight? I was instructed by the duty doctor to sleep with the couple overnight whilst performing 15 min head injury observations! The 'Shack' I had booked on the farm for me and my children was commandeered as an 'Observation' ward. I subsequently slept between the two injured soles which was in itself a strange experience given that they had only been married a week. It was a long night especially as our 'Shack' had no windows and there were constant rustling sounds outside. Heaven knows what was out there. At one point, I felt a thud as something landed on my bed. There was no lighting so I scurried under the sheets hoping that it hadn't been a tarantula or a trapdoor spider. My sleep was further disturbed by some loud howling and screeching noises. My two children decided that sleeping in the Cruiser was a preferable option but not until James had directed the farm staff back to the accident site to collect the couple's remaining bags. He was up most of the night helping. Somehow, we all survived the night albeit worse the wear from lack of sleep. That morning, I was informed that a pack of dingoes had taken down one of the cattle during the night. I and the kids packed up our 4x4 and we continued the last stage of our journey. We were assured that the French couple would be picked up soon. All worked out really well. We met up with them a few days later in Kununurra and they had recovered very well apart from their ruined hire car.

The last place we stayed at before the long drive back to Perth (This time on the highway, not the Gibb River Road) was an Eco-farm. The accommodation comprised of a basic raised solid wooden floor with fly nets as the walls and a tin roof. As it got darker, we could hear strange rustlings again in the surrounding undergrowth. I don't think the netting would have kept much out. After settling in, my daughter went off to the 'En suite' for a wee. I heard the toilet flush then the air was filled with a horrifying scream. She came running out saying that there was something in the toilet after she had flushed it.

James and I tentatively crept up to the loo and sure enough amongst the foam we could also see something moving about but what. I cautiously lifted off the toilet lid only to be greeted by at least 50–60 tiny green tree frogs all desperately clinging on to various bits of plumbing. It could have been a lot worse as the owner of the farm kept pet carpet pythons in his house.

On our travels back south, we had to cross quite a wide river. Good job we had a 4x4 as a smaller car would have almost certainly come aground. Having got across in a dramatic style, with water splashing up the sides of the vehicle, I said to the kids that it would make a great video shot. So, I offloaded Celine with the video camera, positioned her at the side of the river, and then James and I drove back across to the other side. After exchanging hand signals, we set off again trying to make as much splash as we could. We reached Celine who said she'd caught the whole thing on film. Great. Just one problem. Laying barely 3–4 metres from her ankles were five freshwater crocodiles all with jaws wide open. I didn't want to freak Celine so loaded her into the jeep before telling her of her near fate. The rest of the drive back to Perth was long but uneventful.

Even now, 20 years after this great adventure, both my children still reminisce about their wonderful experiences in WA and we all (Luckily) joke about the frogs and crocodiles.

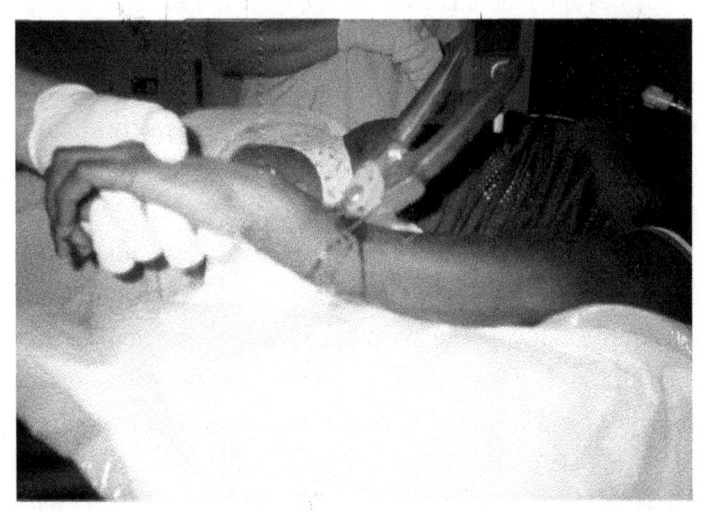

A case of domestic violence.

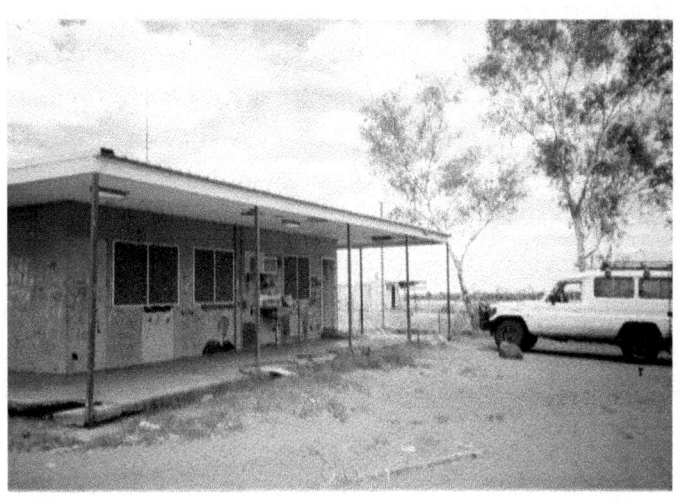

Aboriginal dwelling.

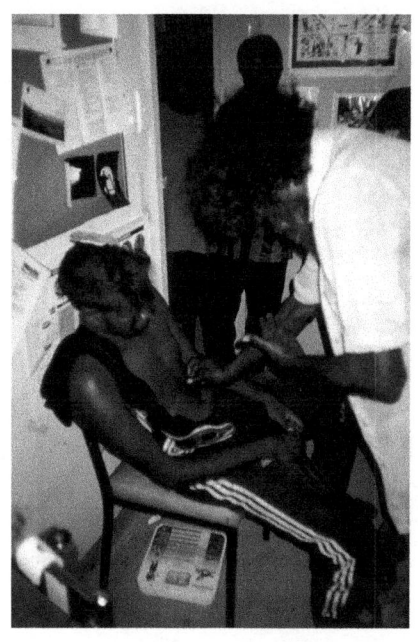

Aboriginal faith healer.

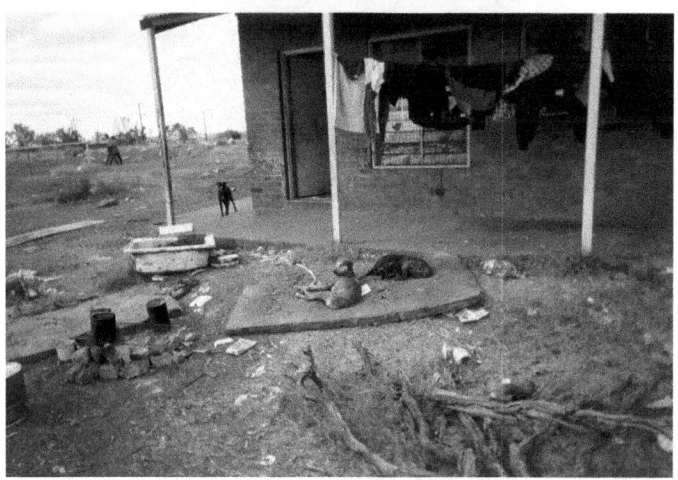

Aboriginal house.

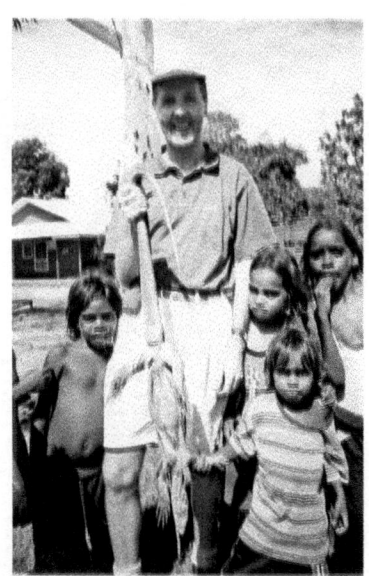

Armed for Bush Tucker.

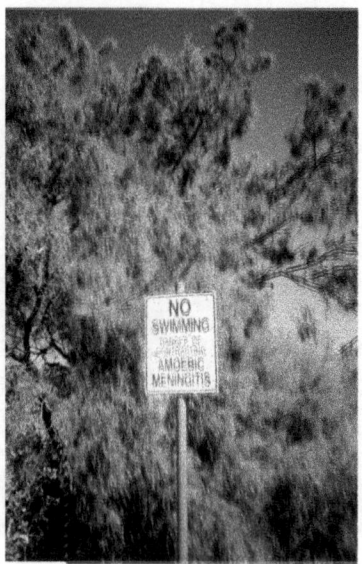

Give that a miss then.

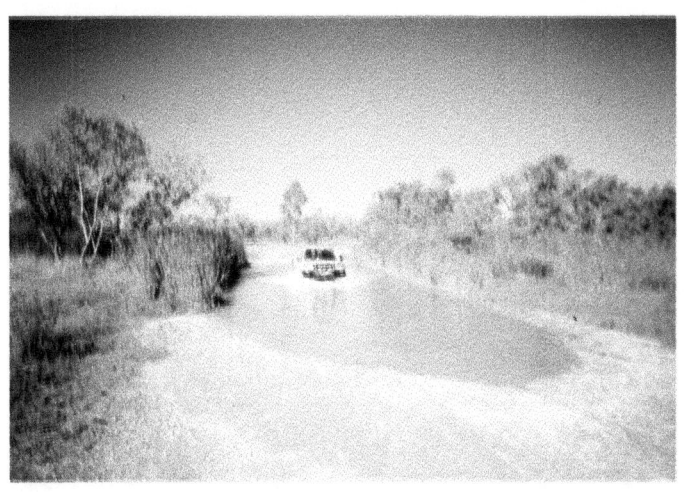

Good job we had a 4x4.

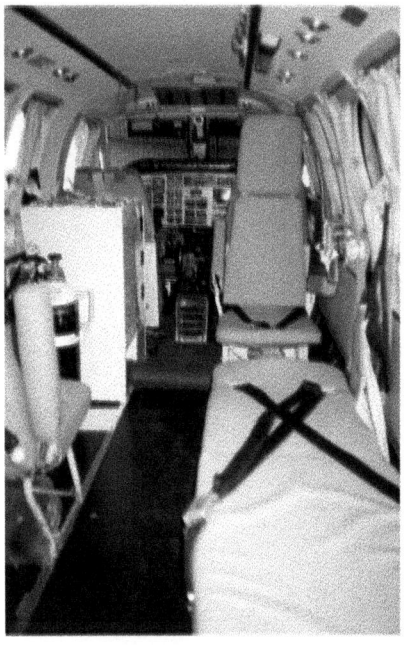

Inside RFDS aircraft.

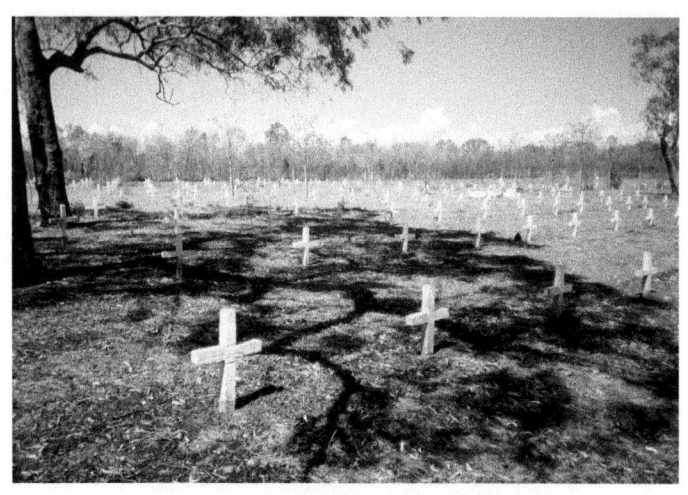

Leprosarium Graveyard, Derby, WA.

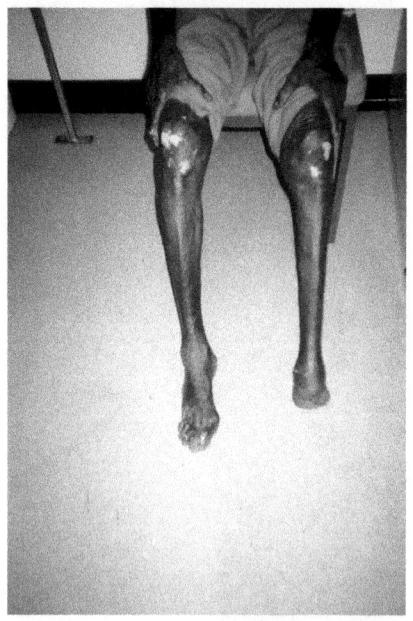

Leprosy.

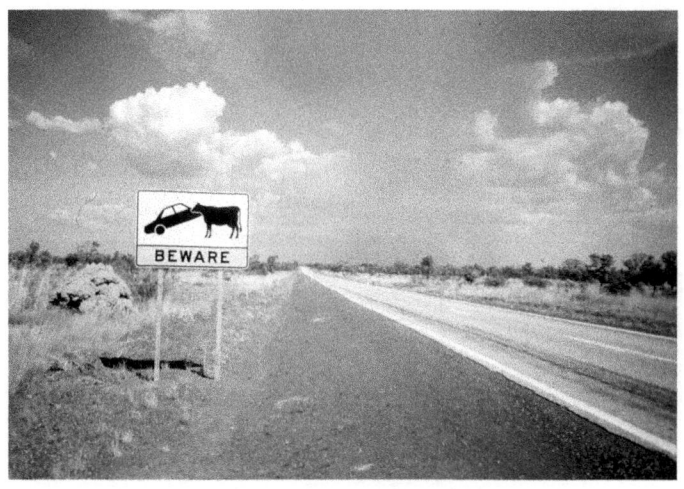

Look out for large cows!

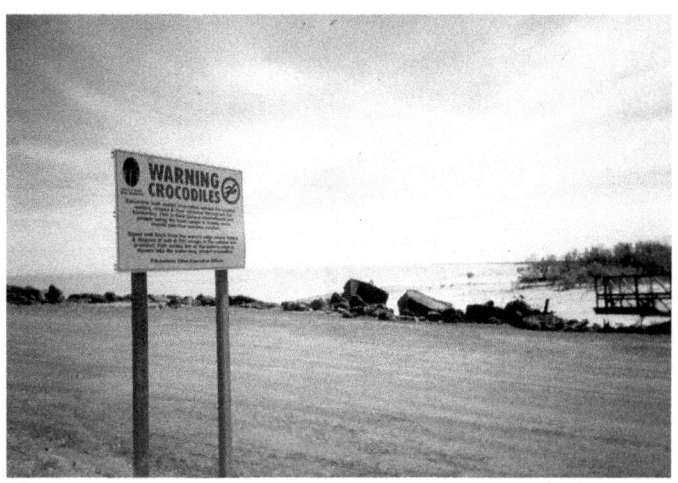

No swimming in the sea then.

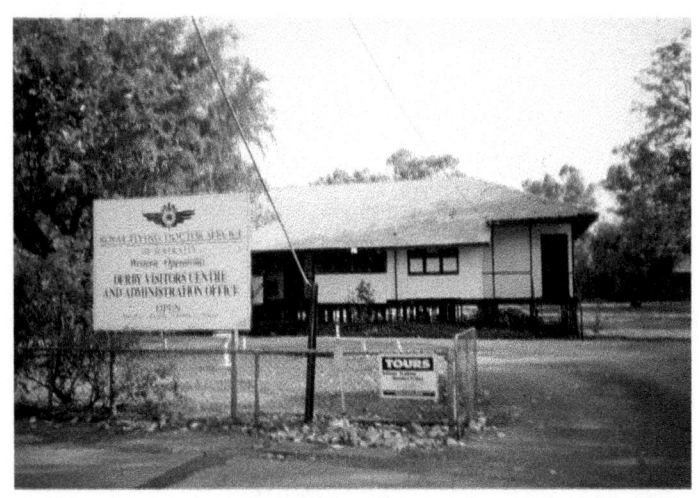

RFD Base at Derby, WA.

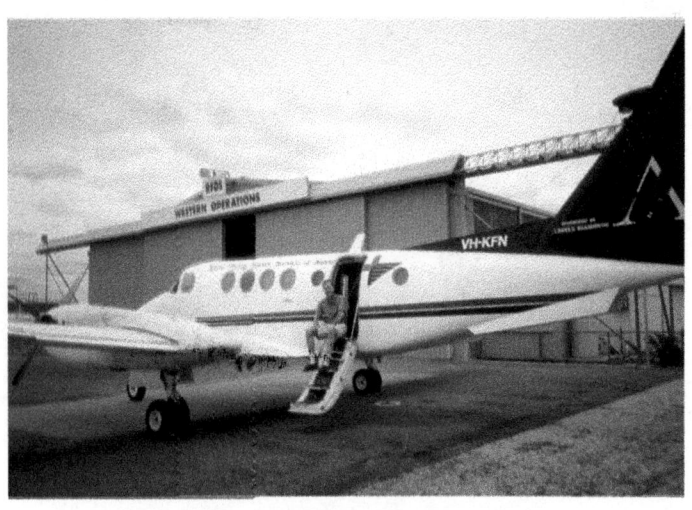

The author's RFDS Base, Derby, WA.

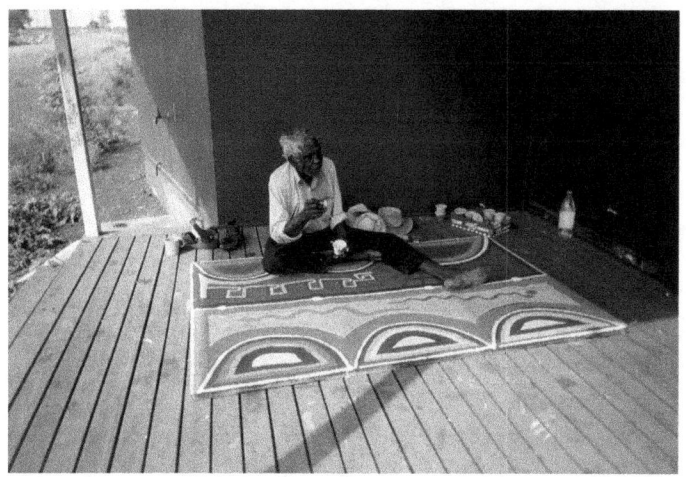

Traditional aboriginal dot painter.

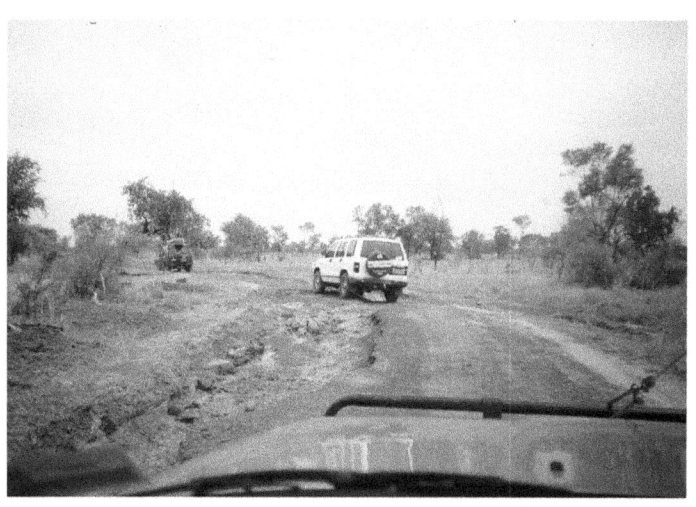

Who said this was the main road?

**If you need to see a nurse or doctor after 4 o'clock then:**

1. come to the hospital and ring the bell
2. A nurse will come to the door and ask you what is wrong.
3. If they think you are not sick, they will ask you to come back in the morning.
4. If they think you are sick, they will let you in. The nurse will try and help you first but if they think you are very sick then they will call the doctor to come and see you.

Only come to the hospital after 4 o'clock if you are really sick.

If you feel sick during the day then please try to get to the hospital before 4 o'clock in the afternoon.

If you have been told you need a dressing done every day then please come before 4 o'clock in the afternoon.

**If you wanna see sista or docta afta 4 o'clock, that mean late aftanoon time or night time, you kin still kam la hospil and:**

1. ringim that bell la thee door.
2. sista will kam and askum you what wrong gatta you.
3. if that sista reckon you not sick, taga sista will tellum you to kam back morning time.
4. if that sista reckon yau sickone, that sista will lettum you la kam in. That sista will helpum you fists but if you propa sickone, that sista will ringimup docta to kam for you la hospil.

You gatta kam la hospil afta 4 o'clock, late aftanoon time or night time only if you propa sickone.

If you feelim sal sickwan day time, you gatta kam la hospil straight away.

If they or doc'a bin tellum you that you gatta kam for dressing ebby day, then you gatta kam eatlytime before 4 o'clock, that mean door bala later aftanoon time or night time.

Aboriginal translation.

# 2000–2004: Back Home – What next?

After returning from Australia, I did some locum GP jobs for a few months back in my old patch in Essex. Whilst sorting all my luggage one day, I came across an old business card of Sue's who I had been seeing some time before my trip abroad. I wasn't even sure that she still worked at the same firm in London. I decided to try and call her. The phone rang and she answered.

"Hi, Sue, it's Peter."

"Peter who?"

"Peter Fowler," I replied. She still seemed perplexed. Eventually, the penny dropped and we started chatting. I told her all about my time in Australia. "Why don't we meet for lunch and I'll tell you more."

"I'm with someone," she said.

"That's fine, it's just a catch up."

We arranged a lunch date and chatted for ages. This was September in 2000. She wasn't 'With someone' as it happens. Over the coming weeks, we met up as often as we could. I was living in rural Essex and Sue had a flat in East Sheen, London. At other times, we phoned each other. During one lunchtime I was doing my home visits, I called in to see an old lady who lived with her daughter. She was very frail and her daughter said that she had been steadily declining all week. I started to examine her chest. It was very bubbly. She was very quiet and pale. At that moment, my mobile rang. It was Sue wanting a chat. I told her I was busy, couldn't talk and would call her back when possible. I cut her off. I still had my stethoscope on the old dear's chest when her heart stopped. She was dead. I've never had anyone die on me under such circumstances. The daughter remained incredibly composed, thanked and hugged me for being there when her mum passed away. It must be awful to have to face that alone. After discussing funeral arrangements, I returned to my car and phoned Sue. Before she could bite my head off, I explained what had happened. I don't think she ever called me at lunchtime again.

Despite this, we got engaged on Christmas Day 2000 and married in September 2001.

Sue was very friendly with a female doctor working in a private practice in the city of London. It just happened that they were looking for another GP, so I got introduced and luckily offered the position. I then spent the next three years there. Our main clients were the big law firms, banks and other city institutions.

Unfortunately, private patients tended to be a lot more demanding than NHS patients, often requesting medication that I would normally not prescribe. Also, some individuals were determined to get their money's worth from a consultation, especially if they'd paid £75 for the privilege. To tell them just to take some paracetamol for their sore throat didn't very often go down very well. There was also a much higher request for 'A specialist's opinion' merely because they had private health insurance (Usually as a work perk). I often felt undermined when 'The specialist' prescribed exactly the same cream for eczema that I would have given. We did, however, have our moments.

On one occasion, a rather short plump male lawyer came in for an appointment. He stated that he had noticed a small lump near his anus, which he then proceeded to describe in minute detail. I asked whether he had used a mirror to gain all this accuracy of detail.

He replied, "No, I used the webcam in my office and had a look at it on the computer screen." For a moment, I envisaged this chap with trousers around his ankles, bending over and parting his buttocks. Thank goodness, his secretary didn't just pop in.

Another young lawyer made an appointment asking for screening for sexually transmitted diseases (STDs). I advised that he should attend a specialist STD clinic (For which there were many in the city area) but he insisted that I do the relevant swab tests and blood tests. I duly took his urethral swab, labelled and bagged it up and sent it off to the lab. The next day I received a phone call from the pathology lab and the specialist there said that there must be a mix-up with the swabs and information as the swab grew Haemophilus influenza (A common cause of upper respiratory infections).

"It was definitely a urethral swab," I confirmed. I managed to get hold of the patient a little later and explained the dilemma. He was not at all concerned.

"I remember now," he said, "my boyfriend coughed when he was giving me a blowjob."

As part of their private health cover, several city institutions had the chance to have annual 'Well person' check-ups. There has always been a lot of controversy as to the value of routine health checks on asymptomatic individuals but many were dead keen and I was totally amazed when some would arrive for their appointment having documented their entire medical history, every blood result, every urine test in colourful glossy flip files complete with flow charts and graphs. The most surprising thing was the men, often quite young, had an expectation for yearly digital rectal examinations of their prostate glands (I'm not quite sure how this originated!). I'm quite sure that there was an open office discussion after one of our clinics there. I can just imagine comments like "And how big did he say your prostate was".

# 2004: Commissioning into the Royal Navy

After two exciting years working in Western Australia, it was quite hard to get back into routine general practice and private medicine didn't really sit comfortably with me. In 2004, the private practice I was working at had a takeover and the new management decided to slim down the medical side of activities. Several doctors would have to go but luckily, I was offered voluntary redundancy which I readily accepted, helped by three months lump sum salary and three years' worth of pension contributions which I readily re-invested.

One day reading through a couple of medical journals I came across a full-page glossy advertisement for the Royal Navy recruiting fully qualified GPs to fill a manning shortage.

Bearing in mind I was 50 years old at this time, I thought that the prospect of being accepted was very slim. I initially contacted the Royal Navy recruitment number in the advert but when I told the chap that I was 50, he just laughed. Thankfully, I managed to get hold of a naval surgeon commander who was working as the medical appointer within the Portsmouth port who offered to meet me for lunch at the HMS NELSON Officer's wardroom. What a grand place this was. I could see myself mingling in here. Having displayed my interest, he suggested that I attend a three-day 'Acquaint' visit at Fort Blockhouse in Gosport where a lot of the medical staff lodged and trained. This was a great eye-opener and enthused me even more. On feeding back to him with my interest, "Good," he replied, "because I've put you down to attend the three-day Admiralty Interview Board (AIB) at HMS COLLINGWOOD in six weeks' time."

On reading up on this, I suddenly felt completely horrified as the three days consisted of a day of written papers, short essays, psychometric and IQ tests, one day of 'Team building' exercises (I never did see the value of building a bridge over a swimming pool just using plastic drums, poles and rope) and the third day of interviews and tabletop practical exercises.

I spent those few weeks studying all about the Royal Navy, visiting as many military museums as I could and actually read several books (As one of the pre-interview questions was to list three books, I had read in the last year ready to discuss at the interviews). I ploughed through several psychometric test books as I hadn't done anything like this for about 30–35 years.

The big day came around very quickly and once at the venue, it was very apparent that I was older than any of the other candidates by a long shot. Day one was a nightmare, the adjudicators handing out questionnaires in quick succession with never enough time to complete (Which I later found out was all deliberate to test individual's response to stress). Day two didn't seem to be much better; running around in groups carrying wooden poles, instructing 'My team' to build this ridiculous bridge over a pool. I recall one of the adjudicators clutching his clipboard commenting to his colleague about my lack of practical skills in building this stupid bridge to which he replied, "But he's a doctor for god's sake, not an experienced marine engineer."

Day three was my high point. I may not have been very bright with the written papers but I don't think any of the others faired any better. I'd hoped by now that they had forgotten about my disastrous bridge-building attempts. Interviews were one-to-one and a more intimidating three-man board of serious-looking senior naval officers dressed up to the hilt in their No.1's complete with gold braid. I was asked no questions directly about the Royal Navy. All that wasted time learning about what ship carried what guns. They did ask me about my book selection and why I had chosen those particular ones. I chose one by John Simpson, the reporter, on his experiences in the Iraq war, one by Rudy Giuliani, the then Mayor of New York City during the 9/11 terrorist attacks, called *Leadership* (I'd had the chance to hear him giving an after-dinner speech in the city earlier that year) and finally, *A tongue in cheek book* by Bill Bryson. Here I felt very at home (Despite not declaring that these were the only books I had read apart from medical ones in years). The final part of day three was a tabletop exercise with three other candidates discussing a scenario about sea currents, ship's speed, fuel consumption etc, none of which meant much sense to me but probably did to the other three, all of whom were probably destined to become engineers or navigators. Given that we were being closely observed by the three wise men, all I could do was to throw in a few intelligent comments hoping that they would feel I had participated at all. At the end of the final interview, I had no idea how I had really done. All candidates were sent into a communal room to await our fate. Shortly after, one of the interviewing officers appeared.

"Dr Fowler, would you please return to the interview room."

My heart was racing. "Congratulations, you are being offered a commission into Her Majesties Royal Navy." Thinking my day was now done, I got ready to leave and go home. But no. "We're getting one of the navy doctors over shortly to do your joiners medical as we want to get you on to the next New Entry Medical Officer's course (NEMO) starting in six weeks' time."

Shortly after, a smart surgeon commodore (1* Brigadier equivalent) appeared and after 'Breathe in/out', a prod and 'Cough', declared me fit to commission. Here was me, an out of work GP suddenly to be appointed as a surgeon lieutenant commander.

The initial six months 'Militarisation' was designed to get all the new recruits in shape for active service. In our troupe were newly qualified doctors, nurses and dentists and a smattering of chaplains, some 25 in all (Usually collectively known as the vicars and tarts). Most of the first four months were based at Fort Blockhouse in Gosport, the former submarine base. Here we learnt military medicine. We had training in gas chambers wearing full protective gear and masks, battlefield emergency trauma care, basic RAF aviation medical care and sea survival training.

As part of the underwater medicine course at the Institute of Naval Medicine (INM) in Alverstoke, we were given the chance to experience going inside a recompression chamber to get a realistic feeling of the type of environment and the effects that divers encountered. These chambers work, in essence by recreating the environment of a dive at depth, then very slowly bringing 'Up' in a controlled manner. This allows the body to do what it should have done in the first place, in order to avoid decompression sickness, often referred to as the Bends. Before entry, we were warned by the instructors that nobody should try this if they had any pre-existing health issues but being hardened military folk by now, we were all for it. During the decompression phase, one chap's tooth exploded and another developed such acute pain in his sinuses that he had to be extracted from the chamber as an emergency. These injuries are caused when air cannot escape from air-filled cavities quick enough, known as barotrauma. Over the years I have seen several burst eardrums from this cause. Some minor ones might heal spontaneously but most are longstanding.

The helicopter escape training was very scary even though I am a confident swimmer and scuba diver. We were strapped into a helicopter simulator then lowered into a deep swimming pool until submerged then we had to open the window hatches to make our escape. Fine I thought, got through that but hadn't realised that we would be doing it all again but this time, in complete darkness and with the simulator being turned 180 degrees upside down. This is the sort of training offshore workers also have to undertake when flying out to rigs in helicopters. It was reassuring that during the helicopter escape training that there were fully kitted navy safety divers within the pool. I didn't think for a minute that the Navy would invest so much into my training just to see me drown! I thankfully avoided ever having to do this again even though it was a requirement before my posting to ARK ROYAL. Having said that, the Captain on ARK did say that he'd never let me fly in a helicopter whilst at sea as he couldn't afford to lose his only doctor on the ship. The

Battlefield Advanced Trauma and Life Support (BATLS) course involved simulated battlefield trauma scenarios using existing war veteran amputees as mock casualties, complete with false blood spurting around. All very realistic. The sea survival training took place on Whale Island in Portsmouth. This incorporated fire-fighting in a mock ship wearing full breathing apparatus and protective clothing. I always wondered after all this what state a ship would be in if its only medical officer was having to do the fire-fighting. Another component included simulations of an engine room of a ship being penetrated by a missile explosion and then slowly filling up with icy cold water and having to repair the damage using wooden wedges and metal props. Finally, we had to jump into icy water in a full thermal suit and swim out to a waiting life raft.

Despite the fact that some of this training seemed quite scary, it did feel like a pleasant break from the purely clinical duties I had been doing for many years previously.

The final two months of militarisation was at the Britannia Royal Naval College (BRNC) in Dartmouth, Devon. This was the most gruelling part of training to date. A man of 50 like me sharing a dormitory with eight other guys was not my idea of fun but of course, at this stage, I was only an officer cadet and would have to wait until passing out parade before I could wear my stripes. Every day started at 6 am with a run around the sports pitch (Not much fun as it was Nov/Dec) then a quick breakfast and on to lectures and demonstrations. There was a lot of romping around in full military kit and rucksacks. We had to run a RN fitness test on our first day here. This is a timed one and a half-mile run and there are set time goals depending on age. I've always hated running but had been practising during the previous few months so would have a go. At the end of the run, the PT instructor called out everybody's name one by one, asked their age and noted their run time. All my younger colleagues had clocked up nine minutes, ten minutes. All passes. He got to me and said, "Time?"

I shouted out 12 minutes 30 seconds.

"Age?" he asked.

"'50, sir," I responded. He looked quite aghast then he scoured his clipboard but there was no 'Pass' time for the over 35s.

He looked up at me and just said, "Bloody good effort."

The training staff seemed to have a thing about 'Beasting' the cadets, pushing them to their limits, which I suppose is not a bad thing when one is trying to prepare them for active military service. One particular day, our troupe was getting fed up with carrying such a heavy load around on exercises so we all decided to empty the two water containers from our bergens (Rucksacks) which would lighten our load by a couple of kilograms and make the march a little easier. Whilst waiting on parade for inspection by the instructors, for some reason that day, they told us to remove our water containers to check that they were full. As one could imagine, seeing that they were all empty we were verbally abused then told to go and fill up our bottles. We had to present these individually to the staff who then casually took them off us and poured the contents of both bottles over our heads. This was followed by 20 imposed press-ups. We didn't try that trick again.

On another day, we felt like we were being 'Beasted' again. We had spent the whole day romping around carrying kit up and down hills and it was a relief to finally make camp in the evening. We only had thin nylon tents but at least it was a refuge from the cold and wind. We had only been in our snug environment for less than an hour when the instructors came around telling us all to break camp, pack everything up and get ready to march off again. We duly did what we were told, marched off then barely 50 yards on, we were told to make camp again.

The staff loved to make fun of us cadets. We had a day learning field crafts; how to improvise on waterproof shelters, how to forage for food and how to build bridges over water (Again). We all got excited when they said they were going to go through the standard ration packs, designed to give each person 24 hours healthy nutrition. But the difference was that we were to be officers. We wouldn't be getting your standard offerings. The instructor had a cardboard ration pack on a table. We all looked in anticipation on what it might contain. He pulled out a small bottle of Bordeaux wine, then a pot of Foie Gras pate, some Fortnum's cheese biscuits, a ready meal of fillet steak with vegetables, a gooey chocolate pudding and finally, a small bottle of single malt whisky. We all looked at each other and couldn't wait to experience such a gourmet meal. Then reality struck home. It was all a co. The actual rat-packs we would subsequently receive had little or no resemblance to what we had been shown and in a blind tasting one would barely recognise what one was eating at all. Mind you, I quite enjoyed the sausage and beans and the chilli boil in the bag meals. I'm sure the pate was actually cat food.

The funniest aspect of life at the college was the military's obsession with order and uniformness. Within our dormitories, we all had to be dressed identically, our shoelaces all had to be tied exactly the same and our pants and socks all had to be folded identically. We even had to iron our bedding and pillowcases with the top sheets folded to specified measurements before each inspection. Our skimpy nylon PT shorts also had to have identically ironed midline creases! The young divisional officers (Younger than my own daughter) conducting the daily 10pm inspections would do a complete sweep of each room and any faults would involve severe actions. If a shirt hadn't been adequately ironed to their satisfaction, they would merely drop it onto the floor. On one occasion, one of the taps in a sink was dripping. Despite it not being our fault that the plumber hadn't managed to fix it, we were the ones to pay the price. Most of the time, we were wearing heavy-duty black military boots. These too were meticulously examined each evening and any minute speck of mud spelt more misery. For some reason, we had to learn by heart all the varied naval knots as if we were a bunch of boy scouts. We were even tested on these during our nightly bollocking. Heaven forbid that we would get a clove hitch wrong.

We were quite lucky as the vicars and tarts that we only had to endure two months at BRNC. All the other poor buggers were there a full year, and many of them were trainee officers from abroad so also had language difficulties. I have to admit that I had never been so fit as by the end of my time there. This was made more apparent when we were fitted for our formal uniforms. The jackets and trousers were 'Off the shelf' which the tailors then chalked up and altered to ensure a proper fit. At the final fitting, I thought that the trousers were a bit too big. I was confidently reassured by the tailor that they would soon fit me just right. How true this turned out to be once we stopped all the exercise and started drinking again.

The time at Dartmouth ended with a four-day field exercise on Bodmin Moor, living in thin floppy tents doing a number of practical command exercises, like building a bridge across a pond only using rope, poles and plastic drums. It's only a pity that I didn't master this at my original commissioning selection. At the end of these tiring four days, we were mustered all together and informed that a helicopter would be landing at a certain map reference in a couple of hours but it would only have room to take about 20 students back to the college. The rest would have to march back (Some five miles) with their full kit. As we had been doing these exercises in groups of six, one of the conditions of being airlifted was that all members of the group had to make the rendezvous together. As soon as the whistle blew, we were off. It was amazing how we found the energy to run up the hills still carrying our kit and rucksacks. It all paid off as our team reached the helicopter site in good time and had an exciting flight back to the college. I did feel sorry for those teams who had some fatties and didn't have a chance of getting there as a group.

The final pass out parade day came. We had spent hours and hours learning to march for our pass out. It was amazingly difficult to get the coordination right. Which arm did one swing with which leg? We shouldn't have spent the night before in the bar as there were quite a few bad hangovers on the day. In fact, of our 'Vicars and tarts' platoon during the parade, two guys had to kneel down to avoid fainting but another actually blacked out and fell straight onto his chin breaking his jawbone in two places. Not quite the exit we had planned for. The parade was inspected by the then first sea lord. As he walked along our line chatting to various cadets, he reached me, took a second look then turned to the commandant of the college and said, "My God, this chaps a bit old. Where are we getting our recruits from now?" He smiled back at me, patted me on the shoulder and moved on. After the ceremony, all the divisional officers that had been our instructors came over to congratulate and salute us. I was now a surgeon lieutenant commander. This was to be the start of a very exciting eight years as a Royal Navy officer.

It was quite an experience doing the whole six-month training. I was now ready to serve. But there was always the question, "What is the best view of Dartmouth Naval College?" Answer: From the rear-view mirror!

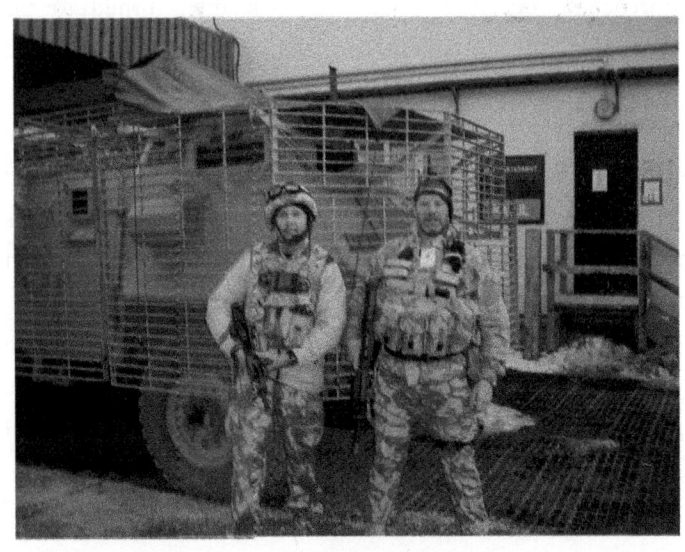

Kabul, Afghanistan with my minder.

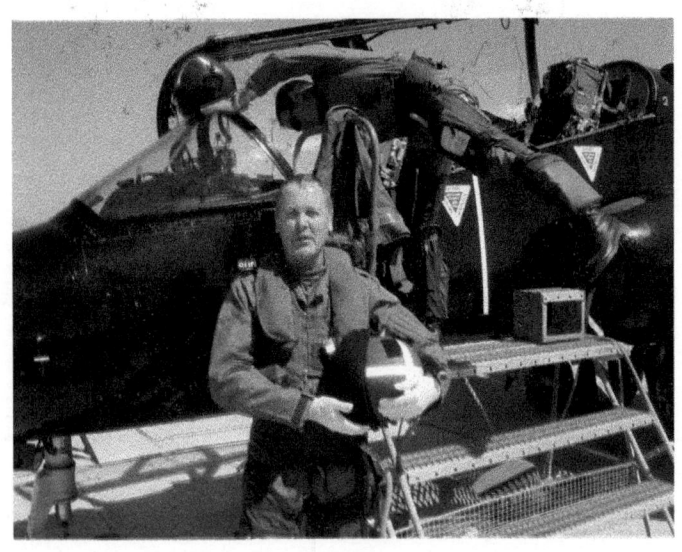

All kitted up and ready to go.

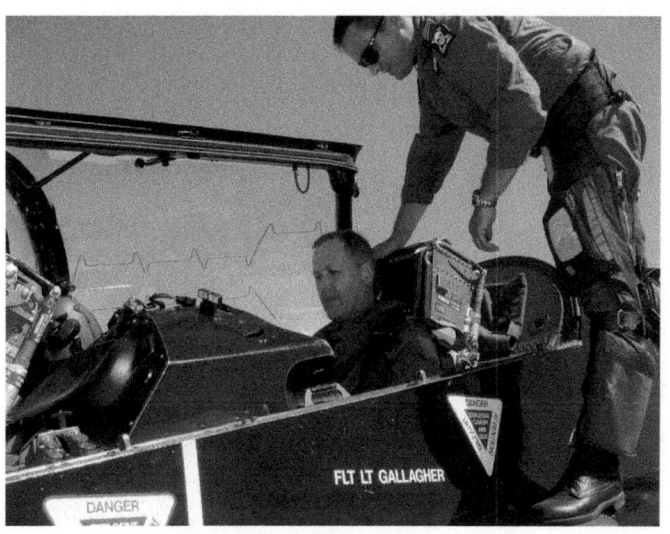

Don't pull that lever – it's the ejector control.

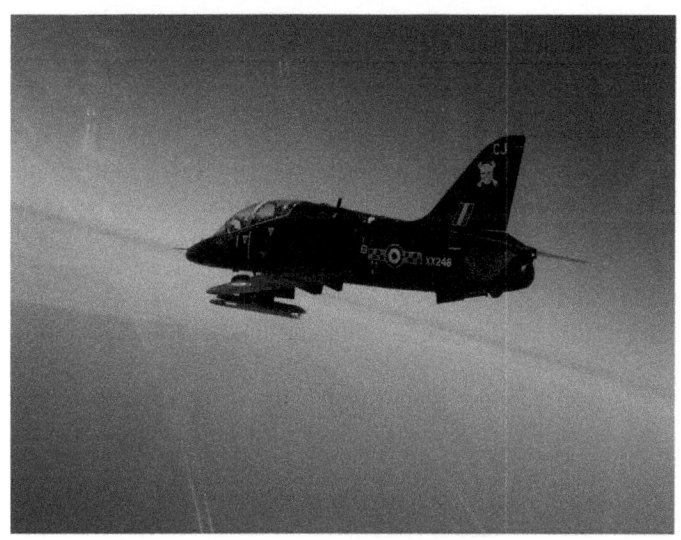

From the cockpit.

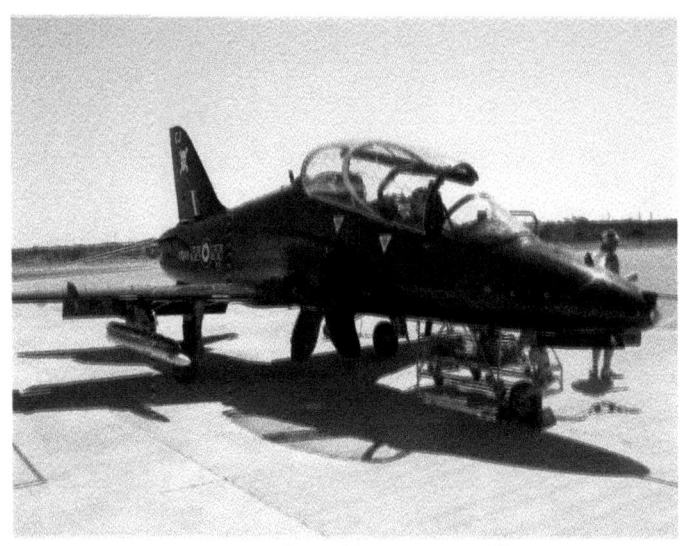

My lift in Cyprus.

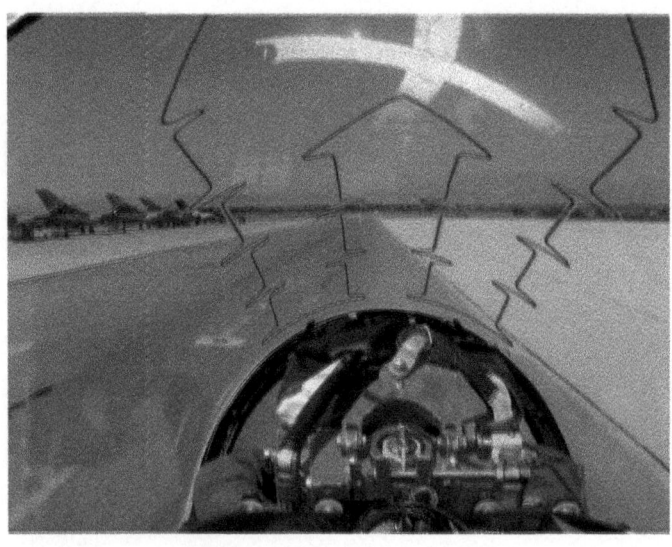

We are off. Note the Tornado jets.

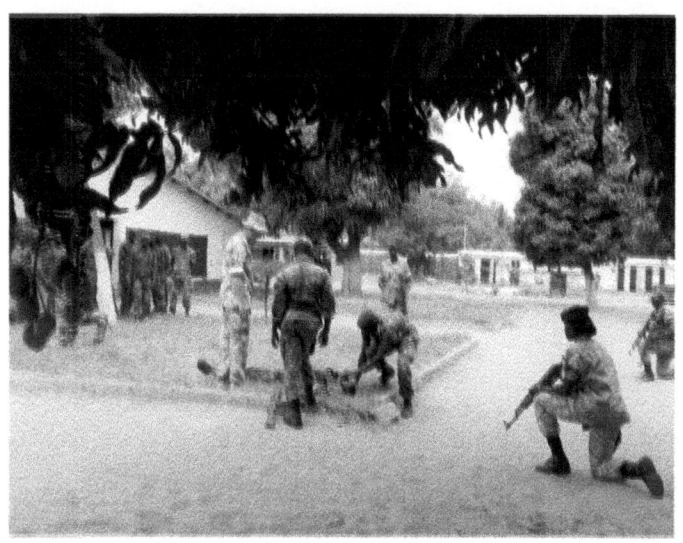

Playing dead for the exercise.

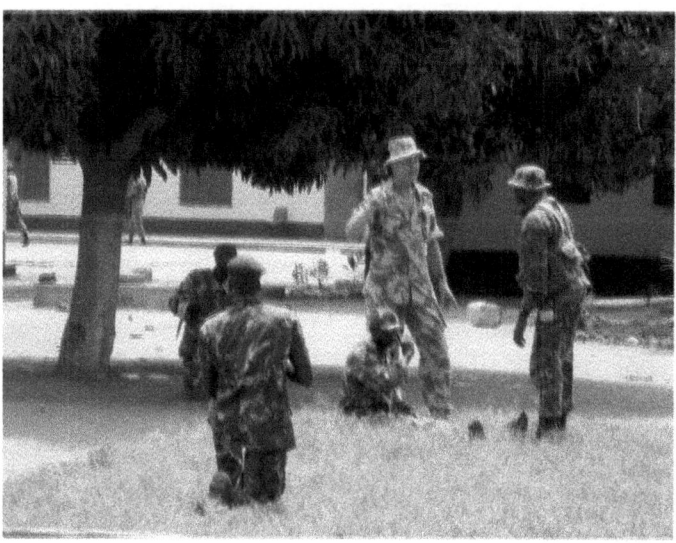

Training the Gambian Army.

# 2004–2012: Royal Navy Medical Officer

It was always a bit of a lottery where one could end up working once in the military although when I had first met the surgeon commander when looking at joining the navy, he had implied that I would be a useful asset to some of the larger military GP practices such as HMS NELSON in Portsmouth which would have suited me fine as easily commutable. How wrong this would prove to be. My first posting was to the Permanent Joint Headquarters (PJHQ) based in North London. Here I was the second officer in command of the medical facility. This seemed like going back to 'Normal' general practice, although we only looked after service personnel and not their dependents. It didn't remain quite so normal though.

My first year there was exciting and varied as I had the chance to spend a month working at the NATO base in Naples. My wife flew out for a few days and we even had a weekend on the island of Capri. I also attended the Trooping of the guard ceremonies in London as part of a military medical team and was on duty on the RFA ARGUS (The Royal Navy's hospital ship) for a week during the 2005 International Fleet Review in the Solent by the Queen.

About halfway through my two years there, I was told that I was required to spend a month in Malawi on a military exercise involving some 100 troops. I and a medical team of army combat technicians were to set up a field hospital and be on duty 24/7 in case of any accidents and injuries. Getting there was quite an ordeal. We were flown by a Hercules transport plane from RAF Brize Norton to Akrotiri, Cyprus which seemed to take forever. We stayed overnight there and re-joined the plane the next day to fly to Nairobi, Kenya. Here we had another night in a hotel until finally, the following day we flew on to Lilongwe in Malawi. Once there, we had to set up our own tents, although thankfully, the engineers had erected some flushing toilets and showers. The thought of having to use a deep dark hole as a loo for a month had horrified me. In contrast, the RAF crew and engineers managed to get their accommodation in a smart hotel in the capital! As our field hospital, we were allocated a rather dilapidated building that in a previous life had been the military airstrip 'VIP' lounge. At least it would suffice if required to bed down any casualties.

The month went quite quickly and I got the chance to spend time with our special forces' troops and even doing some firearms practising. We tried to help the locals as much as we could by distributing pens and paper to the schools and medical bits and pieces to the voluntary run health clinics. It was astonishing to see how many orphans there were whose parents had died of AIDs. Even in the short time we were there, a couple of dozen people died from Cholera.

On a happier note, when we broke up camp to pack and fly home, the army engineers had dismantled all the shower units and toilets and the next thing, dozens of Malawi children ransacked the site and started running off clutching toilet pans and anything else they could carry. Heaven knows what they were going to connect all these items to. Maybe they would just try and sell them on for a bit of cash.

On our last day in Malawi, we noticed a local military lorry carrying a dozen or so military personnel driving across the field near us. One by one, they started jumping off the back of the lorry rolling awkwardly onto the ground. I asked one of our soldiers what they were doing.

"It's the Malawi Air Force doing practice parachute jumps," he replied. "Problem is, they have no aircraft."

Back in the UK, just before the first Christmas at PJHQ, the Colonel in charge of the support unit, our boss, decided that we should all go on a Christmas night out. Someone chose the Medieval Banqueting Halls near the Tower of London. It was decided (Although I don't know by who) that we should all wear fancy dress costumes and given the medieval theme, something applicable. I had never in my 50 years to date ever gone to a fancy-dress event. After much soul searching, I elected to go as Robin Hood. On the day of the night out, we all got changed at the medical centre at PJHQ. I slipped on my brown tights, knee-length leather boots, dainty suede jacket and Robin Hood hat complete with feathers. Once I had my bow and arrows I was set for the evening. We arrived at the Banqueting Halls by coach and piled out onto the street. Just one problem, we seemed to be the only group of revellers wearing fancy dress. Everyone else was in posh suits and city outfits. Not to worry. After a few jars of Mead, who cared. It was a rowdy night but we finally got back on the coach to head home. I was woken by the coach driver. *Where were we?* I thought. There was nobody else on the coach. He had been dropping them all off along the way. I looked out of the window and there was the main gate of PJHQ. The coach driver informed me he had to get back to the bus depot therefore I would have to get off. But I'm dressed like Robin Hood. I cautiously walked up to the main gate where two burly Royal Marine guards were standing clutching their semi-automatic rifles, looking very strangely at me. It was only at this moment that I realised I hadn't taken either my wallet or service ID card with me that evening merely because I didn't have any damn pockets in my tights. I tried to convince the soldiers that I worked at the base as a medical officer but I don't think even I would have believed it had I been in the same position. Eventually, they agreed to call a taxi as I had a married quarter about five miles away. The taxi arrived and an equally stunned-looking Asian chap got out and eyed me over. He did agree to take me home despite having no money on me. Of course, when we got to the house, my door keys were also locked inside the base. By now, it was about 2 am so I started throwing stones at our bedroom window. My wife eventually opened the window and looked equally shocked as even she hadn't seen me in my alternative attire. I have never been to a fancy-dress party since.

One day at PJHQ, I had a young marine come in to see me with conjunctivitis, not an uncommon minor ailment. I prescribed some antibiotic drops and off he went. He returned the next day and his eyes looked even worse, so I changed him to a stronger antibiotic. I couldn't believe it when he returned yet again the next day and his eyeballs looked like someone had been rubbing them in sand. I don't very often take eye swabs but thought that I was running out of ideas so took some and sent them off to the path lab. The next day I received a phone call from the pathologist to say that the swabs had grown chlamydia, that lovely sexually transmitted infection. The following day, three more young marines all walked in together all with identical virulent conjunctivitis. "I think I know what you've all got," I said. It transpired that the four young marines had spent an intimate session with a girl that they had picked up in a nightclub in Watford. I'll let you guess how they caught it! That'll teach them!

A young newly enlisted soldier came in to see me saying that he had a swollen testicle. It had apparently been like that for ages but it was only when he started to have open showers at his military training unit that some of his mates made comments. He had been sexually active for a while, so I asked if any of his partners had mentioned it.

"No," he said. "In fact, they all seemed to comment on my physical prowess."

"Let's have a quick look down there," I advised. He dropped his trousers and hopped onto the couch. My God, I'd never seen such a huge scrotal swelling. It was the size of a couple of small melons. No wonder the girls hadn't complained. He had what is called hydroceles where an abnormal amount of fluid surrounds the testicles. Although he was quite proud of his size, I did refer him to a urologist as he would likely need to have the fluid removed and also further tests to ensure that there was nothing else more sinister occurring underneath.

Another young soldier came in also with 'Tackle' problems. He told me that when he made love with his girlfriend his testicles disappeared up into his groin. It's not uncommon for them to rise a bit but I'd never heard of them disappearing all together, so I started doubting his description.

He then produced his iPhone, pushed the video play button and showed me the screen. There was a graphic image of him mounting his girlfriend, thrusting away, and yes, sure enough, his balls did completely disappear. I'm not quite sure how his girlfriend must have felt having this intimate moment recorded. At least it would save a lot of explanation when he went to the urology clinic to get it fixed (Hyper-mobile testicles are at increased risk of torsion or twisting if not secured within the scrotum).

In the latter half of 2006, I was promoted to surgeon commander. About the same time, out of the blue, I received a call to say that I had been selected to undertake a three-month deployment to Kabul in Afghanistan starting in January 2007. This post was to act as the sole military medical officer at an army base (Camp Souter) on the outskirts of the capital looking after about 450 British, Canadian and French troops. The pre-deployment training itself took about six weeks to complete. This involved full firearms training for a SA 80 semi-automatic rifle and Browning 9mm pistol (Purely for self-defence I was informed). I dreaded to think if I ever had to resort to using them as I wasn't much good on the firing ranges. We had lessons on what to do if captured by the enemy, how to identify booby traps and IEDs and evasion techniques if one of our military vehicles was attacked. We had several war game exercises jumping in and out of land rovers, crawling into ditches firing blanks from our SA80s which all felt like we were having an office away day paintballing. I remained very sceptical about the merits of carrying a credit card sized declaration of the Geneva Convention given to us all which we were advised to show the enemy in the event of being captured. I didn't assume for a minute that it would hold much value.

The big day arrived and my wife drove me to RAF Brize Norton for the military transport to Kandahar, the main airbase in Afghanistan. There was a distinct air of anxiousness amongst the passengers during the flight since this was probably the first deployment to a hostile environment for most of us.

The hardest thing I did before deploying was to write a sealed letter to my wife Sue just in case anything happened to me whilst on tour. I put this with all my personal paperwork but hoped that it would never have to be read.

Once in Kandahar, we had to overnight on bunk beds in a huge prefabricated military building, hundreds of us, until the various units went off to their respective bases and we could fly out the following night under the cover of darkness in a Hercules transporter. This was designed to reduce the risk of being attacked by ground missiles as we approached the city. Although this flight wasn't very long, the worst part was having to wear full body armour and helmet whilst clutching our rifles, which in itself seemed odd given that we weren't given any ammunition! Also, to reduce our visibility to any potential enemy, all normal internal lights were switched off apart from some dim red lights which made everything inside look quite ghostly. As we approached Kabul and had crossed the high mountain range surrounding the city, the aircraft made a dramatic descent into the secure airstrip. It was a bumpy landing but we were all relieved to be on the ground.

We disembarked from the aircraft, collected our kit and walked across to the terminal. It was still dark. The air was freezing cold and misty. Then ahead of me I saw a friendly face calling me over. It was Doug, a larger than life army staff sergeant medic, a Navy Commando, who had been my practice manager at PJHQ and had already been here for the last three months. He looked like the Terminator, about 6'5" tall, built like a wrestler carrying his SA80, about six magazines of ammo and a huge dagger and pistol strung to his belt and an assortment of different smoke grenades strapped to his webbing. After our mutual greetings, he informed me that we just had a 20-minute armoured vehicle journey to the British camp and at that point pulled out and handed me a magazine of ammo to load into my rifle.

The road trip to our base, Camp Souter seemed to take forever. The armoured vehicle had no windows in the back for obvious safety reasons so once again, we sat in complete darkness. To my relief, we finally reached the fortified gates of our home for the next three months. I instantly felt much safer inside.

The base was actually very well serviced. As an officer, I had my own room in a converted warehouse. There was a small officer's mess room and I even joined in with the quiz nights, something I've never done previously. After all, there wasn't much else for entertainment. We couldn't just go off for a stroll around town! I did take a small portable disc player. One of the Afghan tradesmen ran a small kiosk on camp and had a huge selection of films on discs but I did doubt their origins as many looked like they had been filmed from the back of a cinema as frequently the shadow of an individual could be seen walking across the screen. But in the end, it filled some time. All personnel ate in the same canteen, no rank discrimination here. We all wore similar khaki combat uniforms. There were a couple of shops, a huge gym and there was even a weekly market where invited local tradesmen came in to sell their wares. I faired quite well with this as I ended up buying several lovely Afghan silk rugs. My other gem of a find was to purchase four nineteenth century Lee Enfield rifles including a Martini-Henry (Hallmarked c 1876 – Enfield) which was the first breech-loading rifle of the British Army, replacing the previous muzzle loading model and were probably used during the Anglo-Afghanistan wars of the time. Getting them home after my deployment was quite an ordeal, as although the sale of these items was completely legitimate, we still had to go through rigorous security and import documentation. I did cause a bit of a stir with the military customs officers when I finally returned to RAF Brize Norton when they questioned what I had in those four large packages. Luckily, all the paperwork was in order and I was allowed out.

My three months in Kabul was relatively calm, dealing with the usual illnesses and ailments of the 450 odd military personnel within the wire. There was one day when I was walking across a courtyard from my room to take some laundry for cleaning in the main building. I heard a strange sound pass overhead but had no idea what it was. Then suddenly, a voice bellowed out from nearby, "Take cover, sir, that was an enemy missile passing over." We luckily didn't get any direct attacks during my time there although the US base nearby seemed to be hit on several occasions.

The Americans were very keen on 'Hearts and minds' involvement with the local people and they frequently went out to small groups around Kabul to offer medical care and advice but more often just handing out bars of chocolate. The British military was rather against this course of action as they didn't believe it could be sustained or justified. We did agree to go out with the US troops on one occasion but the security cordon required to protect just a few medics did seem disproportionate. It was also sad seeing little toddlers coming to see us requesting lists of medication which was obviously intended for their elderly family members but for which they couldn't source nor afford.

My scariest day was when my team of medics and I were invited to the French Role 3 hospital on the other side of Kabul City for a clinical meeting with other health professionals. This was the main secondary care facility for all deployed military personnel in the Kabul region. Doug had decided that we should go in 'White' vehicles which were less imposing than armoured ones and they would be faster and easier to manoeuvre in a tricky situation. We seconded a couple of Land Cruisers and geared up with all our combat kit including helmet and body armour. Doug told us to fix an ammo magazine for our SA80s. There were strict guidelines when leaving camp. The security guards at the gate would record the time we left and have an estimated time when we should arrive at our location. Driving to the hospital was the first time that I had actually seen anything of Kabul. We must have still stood out like a sore thumb. Two large white 4x4s carrying eight men all wearing quite distinctive military uniforms. Throughout the 30-minute drive, we were constantly observing the scenery and people. I'm sure that 99% of them were innocent civilians but every time we saw a burka-clad person standing on the side of the road, we couldn't help but think, is this a terrorist or suicide bomber?

We got to the hospital OK and had a good day meeting other doctors and medical staff. By about 4 pm, Doug decided that we should head back to our camp as driving in a place like this in the dark would be potentially dangerous. We set off, Doug driving as before. But we found ourselves going up quite a narrow rough road on the outskirts of the city. We didn't come in this way. Then we all noticed up ahead about six square packages neatly positioned across the road. As we slowed down, Doug noticed a dead donkey right on the side of the road. To him, this was a perfect booby trap scenario. I still remember him telling us to unlock our SA80s and prepare for an ambush. I wished then that I'd paid more attention to my ambush drills during pre-deployment training. The road was so narrow that Doug couldn't just do a three-point turn and every minute we were stationary put us at a potentially increased risk of being attacked. Eventually, we managed to get the vehicles turned around and hastily made our way back to the hospital and safety. We reported the incident to the CoC there and shortly after, they deployed a rapid response team in armoured vehicles to the site where we had located the packages. Sure enough by then, they had all disappeared. Was it just kids trying to intimidate the enemy, we'll never know?

We were now desperate to get back to our base. Thankfully, we were given an armed escort to the outskirts of Kabul and told just to follow the road around the foothills and it would take us back to our camp. As if the day hadn't been eventful enough, we then passed a landscape difficult to describe. It was what is known as the Russian Tank graveyard. Strewn over acres and acres of snow-covered fields were literally hundreds of rusting tanks and other armoured vehicles left by the Russians in 1989 after their disastrous war with Afghanistan.

Unfortunately, I didn't get a chance to take any photos as our priority was to get home. We seemed to be driving through the graveyard for ages but just then we spotted what looked like a roadblock up ahead. There were barriers across the road and several military vehicles parked nearby but we were unsure who would be running a roadblock in the middle of nowhere. Once again, Doug told us to unlock our SA80s just in case. We drove up to the barrier and several uniformed soldiers approached us. In broken English, they asked to see our ID cards. They were obviously happy with this, opened the barrier and let us pass through. Thankfully, they were Afghan troops. The rest of the journey was uneventful and we safely arrived back at our camp. In the remaining few weeks in Kabul, I never left the camp again.

In the three months in Kabul, I didn't really have to deal with anything too dramatic apart from one young soldier who sustained a rifle wound to an arm. We never did find out whether this was accidental or self-inflicted as we got him down to the hospital soon after the incident.

Life in the camp was aided by the sending and receiving of mail in the form of 'Bluies' (Like the old airmail letters) from home and regular parcels from friends and family, full of snacks and chocolate. Internet use was very restricted for obvious security reasons. We did receive credits to use a satellite phone briefly each week.

I wasn't sad to leave. I'd in effect been on sole doctor duty 24/7 for the whole three months. As we were driven back to Kabul airport by armoured vehicle, I just hoped and prayed that having got through all this time unscathed that we wouldn't come a cropper at the last hurdle. When the doors opened, we were within the fenced airfield. There was now just the Hercules flight back to Kandahar to meet our homeward aircraft.

On return to the UK after such a deployment, we were all allowed a welcome post-deployment leave period which felt very strange and unreal since I had spent the last three months walking around in full military attire with a machine gun. I couldn't help but feel privileged to have served in an operational conflict abroad. The icing on the cake was to receive my Afghan deployment medal which acts as a permanent reminder of my active service abroad.

My wife and I met up with Doug sometime later where he reiterated to her that he would have given his life to protect me during the deployment. I truly believe him, a real hero and soldier.

By the time I had returned to PJHQ after my well-deserved leave, I received a phone call from the navy doctor's 'Appointer' who allocates successive postings. He politely suggested that I would like the chance to work in Cyprus. This would be as the senior medical officer in the Episkopi Garrison, which is part of the Sovereign Base Areas, and governed by the UK.I had to call my wife to get her thoughts on the matter but thankfully, this posting was accompanied i.e. family could go as well, so it was easier to sell. Luckily, she agreed and soon we were packing up household items to ship out. It was to be just over a two-year posting. We had a comfortable if not a very dated married quarter but it was on a patch where a lot of senior officers lived including the Commander of British Forces, senior police officers, the judge, the dentist and vicars. We could walk to the beach in a lovely cove within 15 minutes. Many a beach party was had!

General practice in Episkopi was much like that in the UK as we looked after all the military and the dependents of service personnel. We also oversaw the hundreds of troops returning from Iraq and Afghanistan post-deployment who came into Cyprus for a short period of 'Decompression'. Here for most of them, this was their first time in possibly six months that they could relax and unwind before returning to their families in the UK. They were also given various briefs by staff on how to deal with PTSD and other possible psychological problems once back into the real world.

What made the role of doctor more interesting was the fact that we acted as the first responders to acute incidents whether it be RTAs, swimming accidents, even unexplained deaths. To fulfil this role, we had to undertake driver training for emergency vehicles that used blue lights and sirens. That was quite good fun. The senior medical officers were also appointed as deputy coroners to support the sole judge within the Sovereign Base.

Whilst on duty one day, I received a call to attend a casualty at one of the local beaches. On arrival, there were a crowd of people trying to administer CPR to a middle-aged man who had been found floating face down in the sea. He had apparently been out in the bay on a jet ski and it was only when this was found grounded on the beach that they came across the body. It later transpired that he was not wearing a life jacket, had not engaged the kill-cord of the machine and couldn't swim. I declared him dead at the scene and he was taken away by the RAF sea rescue helicopter to the military hospital at RAF Akrotiri.

About the same time, a couple of young children came across the remains of a man at the bottom of one of the cliffs near the married quarters. There wasn't much flesh on the torso but then there was a colony of vultures nesting nearby. Post autopsy, I had to authorise the disposal of the body as the judge was in the UK at the time.

The social life at camp was amazing. Due to the very pleasant weather, many events could be conducted outdoors throughout the year. Most were quite formal occasions wearing full military attire. We often had visiting military bands to perform at these. I was pinged to be the President of the Mess Committee (PMC) for six months, not a role I really enjoyed as it meant having to oversee mess functions and I hated speaking publicly but it was a good tick in the box (Not that I had much choice to refuse!). On one Trafalgar night dinner, I managed to secure a leading surgeon rear admiral to fly out to Cyprus, give a memorable after-dinner speech about Lord Nelson, then fly back to the UK the next morning.

One of the highlights of my time in Cyprus was when I received a phone call one day asking if I would be interested in going out for a flight in a Hawk trainer jet. I didn't have to be asked twice. The next day I drove over to RAF Akrotiri and after a full briefing induction (Including how to conduct myself in the event of being ejected from the cockpit) donned the full pressure suit, applied the mask and helmet and off we went. It was an amazing hour flying around the southern coast of Cyprus at 600 mph, experiencing G-force and even taking controls for short times. Several days after this, a Harrier jump jet carrying a young RAF airman on a similar 'Jolly' had an engine failure and the two occupants had to eject. Luckily, both were unscathed, more than one can say for the £50m Harrier!

Also at this time, the Red Arrows RAF display team did their pre-season training in Cyprus as the flying conditions were so good. We witnessed a number of displays and had the opportunity to meet all the pilots on several occasions.

At the beginning of our third year in Cyprus, I was asked if I would extend my posting there another year or so but we felt that it was the time to return to the UK. We had bought a house in Hampshire whilst away and wanted to get back to take more control of refurbishments. It was now early 2010. To my complete surprise, the appointer asked if I would be interested in joining HMS ARK ROYAL, the navy's flagship Aircraft Carrier, as a senior medical officer. This was an amazing opportunity as a naval doctor as it was the only surgeon commander's sea posting at that time. There was just one problem. I had not previously served on any other naval ships apart from a week on RFA ARGUS, the navy's hospital ship, moored in the Solent during the Queens Fleet review (So not a particularly testing experience) and I was a bit unsure how my sea legs were. I managed to arrange both a week at sea on RFA FORT GEORGE (A Fleet Auxillary vessel) and HMS ILLUSTRIOUS, another carrier, so I wouldn't appear quite so naive when I finally boarded ARK.

I was the sole doctor on board but had a team of naval medics and a dentist. The ship had a total complement of about 1,000 personnel including a Harrier squadron, various helicopters and all their support crew.

The hardest aspect of living on a warship was the fact that unlike a cruise ship with its grand staircases and atriums, the whole ship was divided into multiple smaller compartments separated by heavy lockable metal doors, designed to minimise damage during any possible assault such as a fire or missile attack. There were no elaborate stairwells, just metal ladders. To get from one end of the ship to the other, involved going up and down multiple decks, zigzagging across the ship. I initially got completely lost many a time. It must have seemed odd that someone of my rank would repeatedly have to stop and ask a junior rating which was the front and back (Sorry, I mean bow and stern).

There were about 100 Officers aboard ARK, many training for their various speciality careers such as marine engineering, weapons, logistics and navigation. As the medical officer, I was part of the command group who usually met twice daily for briefings on the weather, flying activities for the day and any update regarding security threats. Meals on board were invariably very good considering the logistics of stocking so much produce for 1,000 personnel. Historically, the captain ate alone most of the time at sea. I was lucky enough though to be invited to have dinner with him several times, sitting on the bridge seeing the bow of the ship rise and fall as the sun set.

As officers, we were lucky enough to have our own cabin, albeit 'Compact' with a couch that transformed into a very narrow bed at night. Cot sides were provided to prevent one from falling out of bed during rough seas. Mornings started with one of the stewards knocking on the cabin door presenting a mug of tea at 7am. Our laundry was miraculously collected during the night and the freshly cleaned uniforms were delivered back the next morning. Likewise, our heavy-duty work boots were 'Bulled' to perfection every day. Junior ratings had far less in the way of comforts and had to endure accommodation messes of up to 30 individuals, stacked like sardines in a can.

I had to fly out to Halifax, Nova Scotia, to meet ARK where she was attending the Canadian Navy's centenary and the Queen did a fleet review. I must say that she looked quite small moored up against a gigantic US helicopter assault flat top. Here I received a handover from another naval doctor before he returned to the UK. We even had David Cameron come and give us a morale boosting speech on board, although this would prove a false premise in the weeks to come. After a few days in Halifax, we set sail south towards Florida. This would take about 28 days during which we didn't see any land.

During these days at sea, the crew were subjected to regular 'Emergency drills' to keep everyone on the ball. This included mock man overboard scenarios, mock crashes on deck and mock fires in the engine rooms. During these days, the Harriers would regularly fly off the ramp for training exercises. They always looked a bit ungainly taking off. To aid in getting the right elevation to take off, the ship had to be cruising at a specific speed into an oncoming wind to gain enough uplift. It was always amazing seeing them vertically descent onto the flight deck of a moving ship. By now, their fate had already been signed as they were assigned to history on this very last major voyage. From the captain's bridge, I watched the last Harriers ever to take off from an aircraft carrier. It was very emotional as they flew back over the ship information, wings tilted for their last ever flypast saluting the ship that had supported them all these years.

One morning I was doing a routine surgery (If you can call doing a clinic on a moving aircraft carrier routine) a young sailor came in having noticed a few bruises on his shins and thighs. He was quite well in himself and I just assumed that he had probably banged himself on any number of metal doors, ladders and bulkheads. I asked him to keep an eye on things and to return if any more developed. Sure enough, the next morning he returned, now with even more bruises all over with no obvious mechanisms of injury. ARK had very limited medical equipment on board. There were no X-ray facilities. An ECG machine would not work whilst the ship was moving due to the continuous shuddering of the vessel. But we did have a very basic blood test machine. I got my lab technician to run a full blood count and when the results printed out it said that his platelet count was 10,000. The normal range is 150,000–450,000. We assumed that the results were false, so we recalibrated the machine, left it a few hours then rechecked. Same result 10,000. His white cell count and haemoglobin were normal which suggested that there was no bone marrow failure. From my hospital days way back, I wondered if this could be Immune Thrombocytopenic Purpura (ITP). The worry here was that platelets help the blood clot by clumping together to plug small holes in damaged blood vessels. If he were to injure himself, he could bleed to death.

I informed the captain that we needed to get the lad transferred to a hospital ASAP. Shortly afterwards, a helicopter was deployed to take him to a military hospital in Virginia. I spoke to the treating physician the next day who confirmed my initial diagnosis. Not bad I thought. They gave him various drugs including steroids but were unable to get his platelet count any better. Eventually, he was transferred back to the UK for further treatment. I met up with him a few months later at a naval medical centre back in the UK. His platelets never improved beyond 50,000 and he was deemed unfit to continue military service so was medically discharged.

Before the ship had even reached Cape Canaveral in Florida for a well-deserved R&R for the crew, the UK government declared that ARK was to be decommissioned in 2011. This also meant the demise of the sea-going Harriers.

After two weeks in Florida, ARK once again started her 12-day crossing back to Portsmouth in the UK, accompanied by a support RFA supply ship, a Type 42 Destroyer, HMS Liverpool, and a submarine.

We were nearly 200 miles off the US coast when I received a phone call from another Navy doctor on one of our support ships. She had only joined the ship in Florida and this was her first sea posting. She was concerned about one of her crew who she was concerned might have had a stroke as he was complaining of severe headaches and high blood pressure. The options were to send a helicopter over to the other ship and fly him back to ARK but then I had no specialist equipment to do any investigations, or me to fly over to the other ship. This was not allowed as I was the only doctor on ARK and if anything happened to me, the 1000 crew would have no medical cover. The last option was to send one of our helicopters, pick up the patient and fly him back to a military hospital in Florida. The captain of ARK agreed to the latter option but because we were already about 200 miles from shore, we had to turn the whole convoy around to get into a near enough flying distance for the helicopter. In the end, the captain ordered two helicopters for the pickup for safety reasons. So, both each flew a 400-mile round trip to deliver the patient. I called the hospital the following morning for an update on our patient and was informed by the treating doctor that they had diagnosed a migraine attack! I informed my captain who tutted then started scribbling on some paper. "Peter," he said, "when you add up all the extra costs in fuel for the ships and the deployment of two helicopters and crew, this little exercise has cost the military £300,000." I was politely reminded that the 20,000 Ton ARK used a gallon of fuel every six inches. The sailing back home was very relaxed. There were fancy dress competitions (Why would someone take a spiderman costume on tour?) BBQs and even deck sports, although we lost a fair few basketballs overboard. One naval chap even ran the length of a marathon around the flight deck! There was even the chance to do some clay pigeon shooting. I thoroughly enjoyed firing the Gatling gun at a target being pulled along behind the ship.

In the evenings in the calm Atlantic waters, one could often see dolphins and whales in abundance, lying motionless on the flat sea surface.

Once back in port, it was then the time to start her preparation for scrapping. As a final farewell, she sailed up to the western coast of Scotland to off-load all her ammunition, then sailed around the north of Scotland to Newcastle, where she had been built, for the local people to see her for the last time. As we sailed around the north of Scotland, we hit a heavy gale force, so rough that the waves were crashing over the flight ramp. I'm usually quite good at sea but on this occasion, all I could do was lie on the floor and pray for the storm to end. A final 'Run ashore' in Hamburg completed ARK's 25 years serving the Royal Navy. The biggest pity and disappointment was that we sailed into Portsmouth harbour for our final entry on the 3 December, 2010 but the weather had been so bad that a lot of the crew's families including my wife couldn't get there to see her come in. It was a very proud moment though, standing on the bridge with the captain and other senior officers, seeing the whole ship's crew standing to attention along the sides of the ship and hearing the applause from the crowds on shore as we passed.

Prior to the news of ARK's decommissioning, arrangements had been made for the Queen to attend its 25$^{th}$-anniversary celebration in Portsmouth. It had been assumed that she would not attend due to the change in circumstances but she insisted on coming. On the day, my wife and I had the privilege of meeting her face to face and having a short chat. All the officers had to remove their ceremonial swords for the presentation just as a precaution.

Whilst in Portsmouth, I continued to work on the ship until April 2011 when the last members of her crew disembarked. I was due to leave the navy in April 2012 and thought that the appointer might give me some time off on gardening leave as time was getting short but oh no, I was posted to Gibraltar for six months. Not only that but the first month of this posting was to be in the Gambia as the medical officer to a training team from the Royal Gibraltar regiment, helping the Gambian Army and Police force.

One of my responsibilities on arrival in the Gambia was to assess the medical facilities just in case one of my soldiers became ill or injured. We were introduced to an army Colonel who was in charge of the military hospital in Banjul. This proved to be quite an eye-opener. They only had a basic chest X-ray machine; all the other specialised equipment was broken. They had so few surgical instruments that they 're-sterilised' them for the next operation (Even assuming that the steriliser worked). The wards had shutters but no windows, opening on to an open courtyard that had a stagnant stream running through it. One could see the malarial larvae squirming about quite easily. The beds only had any bedding if a patient's relatives brought some in, otherwise, it was just a plastic bed cover and the hospital didn't provide any meals for the inpatients. Again, the relatives had to bring this in. I even saw people cooking meals on small primus stoves next to the beds!

In contrast, we were taken to a medical research council hospital in the same town which was clean and airy, where all the staff wore pristine white coats and the beds were immaculate. This hospital was obviously funded by international money. They were doing a lot of research on infectious diseases, especially malaria. The lead doctor offered to show me around the wards. There were about 20 inpatients at the time. The diagnoses he reeled off sounded like an extract from a tropical disease book. One had cerebral malaria, another meningococcal septicaemia, another tuberculosis and several other diseases that I'd never even heard of. The hospital had very limited supplies of medication and quite often their patients didn't present until quite advanced. I returned to the hospital at the end of our month there as we had some drugs and sterile dressings which we couldn't take back to Gibraltar, so I donated them. The wards seemed incredibly quiet. There were no inpatients. I was going to congratulate the senior doctor on his success in treating all of the patients. He then turned to me to say that all of them had died.

We were fortunate to be put up in a beachfront hotel. This was however a sharp contrast to how the Gambian soldiers lived. We had a chance to look around their camp and their married quarters which comprised of flimsy tin shacks where often 6–8 individuals would sleep. The ablutions consisted of dank toilet blocks riddled with flies and lizards. The families were very basically dressed, children didn't have any footwear and many a soldier was wearing non-matching boots. Few seemed equipped with usable weapons, most practised drills with broom handles.

After this eye-opening view of how the Gambians lived, we passed a group of about eight soldiers crouched around a giant metal caldron some four feet across balanced on a huge open fire. Within the pot, we could make out numerous fish heads and bones, some meat like shapes and an assortment of vegetables. As the various soldiers dipped their hands into the pot squelching a handful of solids and consuming it directly, any surplus fluid seeping back into the pot, they turned to us and asked if we wanted to join in with their meal. I looked up to the nearby ablution block remembering that there was no running water there, and politely declined.

My remit was to teach the Gambians basic field first aid and trauma management. Easier said than done. As for example, when I asked how they would treat a snake bite, the consensus was for them to gouge out the venom with a knife. How would they treat a burn? Apply toothpaste was the answer. How would they treat intestinal parasites and worms? Wait for it; get the patient to drink paraffin. I had my work cut out. Trying to teach them some trauma scenarios, I asked one of the female soldiers to lie on the floor with a simulated puncture wound to her chest from a bullet. I had gone over this management in the classroom but this was their chance to show the practical treatment. I told the other soldiers what the scenario was and asked them to treat the injury. They all just stood around the 'Wounded' girl doing nothing.

"Why aren't any of you applying pressure to the wound and checking her airway?" I asked.

"Because we are all Muslim men and it is forbidden to touch a woman unless we are married." I did try to instil that we were all soldiers and that we had a duty to care for our wounded colleagues but obviously, different cultural beliefs and teaching prevailed.

Another 'Practical' scenario I organised didn't prove to be much better. One of my Gibraltar soldiers had managed to obtain a long bone from a local butcher that he dressed in some scraps of meat, placed in an old army boot and generously coated it in tomato ketchup. We then got one of our guys to lie in a field and scream out that he had been blown up by a mine. My Gambian soldiers were instructed to find the soldier and assess and treat any injuries. On seeing the 'Amputated' leg, two of them vomited and two blacked out. I just hope that the Gambia is never invaded by an enemy.

Thankfully, my group of soldiers remained very healthy during our month here. That was apart from one day when several of them presented to me complaining of multiple large abscesses on their backs and buttocks. I initially thought that these had been triggered by the humid heat combined with these guys wearing full combat clothing. But one of the soldiers decided that it would be a good idea to puncture one of these huge boils. To his disgust, out slithered a one-centimetre long maggot. Of course, the others had to follow suit and low and behold, out of each boil yet more of these aliens squirmed out. I had no idea what on earth these creatures were so went and spoke to a local pharmacist. I was informed that these were typical maggots or grubs from a Bot fly. The problem had been that my soldiers had been hand washing their combats and then leaving them to dry overnight on the balcony rails. Apparently, not what one does in places like the Gambia because the Bot flies lay their eggs on moist warm surfaces which then change into larvae and worse of all, these then burrow into the skin. One can starve the larvae of air by applying Vaseline or something else similar over the abscess which causes them to burrow out but as one could imagine, soldiers did not have the patience to wait for nature to act so resorted to the knife.

Back in Gibraltar, I was the duty doctor on one occasion when I received a call from the main hospital requesting our help dealing with a diver with a possible decompression injury as the only decompression chamber nearby was within the Royal Navy harbour and manned by the military. I have to admit that during my previous navy years, I had undertaken several underwater medicine courses and even experienced being in a decompression chamber but never had to deal with such a case myself. I went to the hospital to see the patient, a commercial diver who had been cleaning the hulls of some ships in the harbour but who had exceeded his dive times. When he ascended, he developed severe pain in one of his shoulders. The hospital staff had done bloods and X-rays all of which were normal so assumed that a decompression illness (The bends) was most likely. We transferred him to the dockside chamber and conferred with the naval underwater specialist back in Portsmouth who recommended that we go ahead. Thankfully, one of the navy technicians volunteered to stay in the chamber with the patient whilst they recompressed him. Amazingly, within two minutes of starting this, the patient's pain had disappeared. They remained in the chamber for about six hours until all the gases had stabilised then they could bring him out. Thank goodness, I didn't have to endure it.

Just before I left Gibraltar, I was requested by the Commander of British Forces (CBF) to attend a function within the naval base to meet the then Defence Secretary, Liam Fox.

As he went around the line of gathered officers and officials, he was introduced to me as the senior military doctor there. He asked me how long I'd been posted there.

"I shouldn't even be here," I said. "I was the surgeon commander on our Flag Ship, HMS ARK ROYAL until you recently decommissioned her." He suddenly looked a trifle embarrassed then quickly shuffled off to the next in line.

In the course of writing this book, I looked through a couple of cardboard boxes of photographs and other paperwork from the attic left after my mother died but which I hadn't got around to perusing. With all the anniversaries of the world wars recently, I started to investigate if any of my family had had any military experience. As already mentioned, I never really knew my father and my grandfather never ever spoke about the wars when I was young. He did recall once telling me how the V1 doodlebugs used to fly overhead during WW2. There was apparently only panic when their engines cut out meaning they were coming down and it was time to head to the shelters. From my research, I was amazed to find out that my grandfather actually served in the Royal Navy during WW1 as a rating on HMS Phaeton, a light cruiser and later a minelayer seeing action in Jutland and the Dardanelles.

My mother served with the Auxiliary Territorial Services (ATS); I believe working in a secretarial role and attained the rank of Sergeant. I came across a commendation letter she received at the end of WW2 for her contributions to the D-Day invasion. She had never discussed this throughout my childhood.

The only information about my father was that he served in the Tank Regiment (A Desert Rat) in WW2 and saw action in N. Africa. I believe that his tank was blown up causing him hearing problems and he had to leave the army as a result.

Finally, my uncle served in the Canadian Navy during WW2. He married my mum's sister after the war but both have been dead for a number of years now, so I'll never know the whole story.

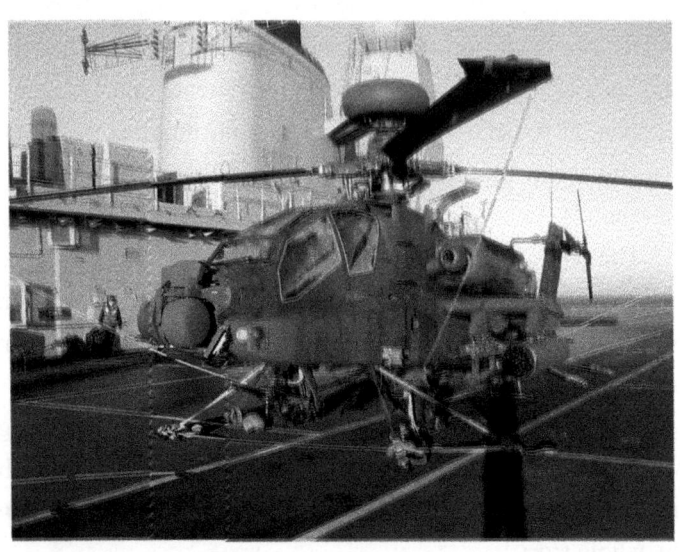

Apache attack helicopter.

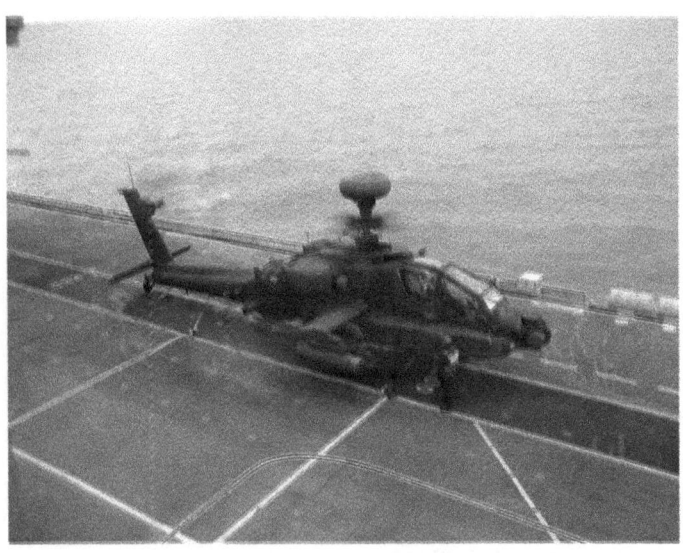

Apache ready to take off.

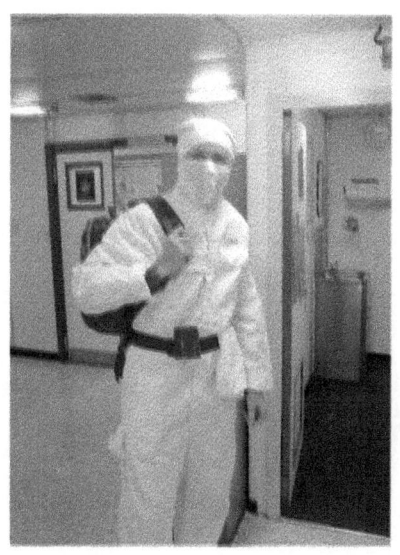

Author in 'flash' suit during exercise.

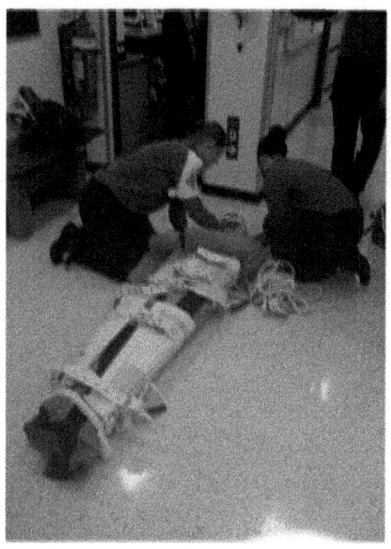

Casualty simulation on ship.

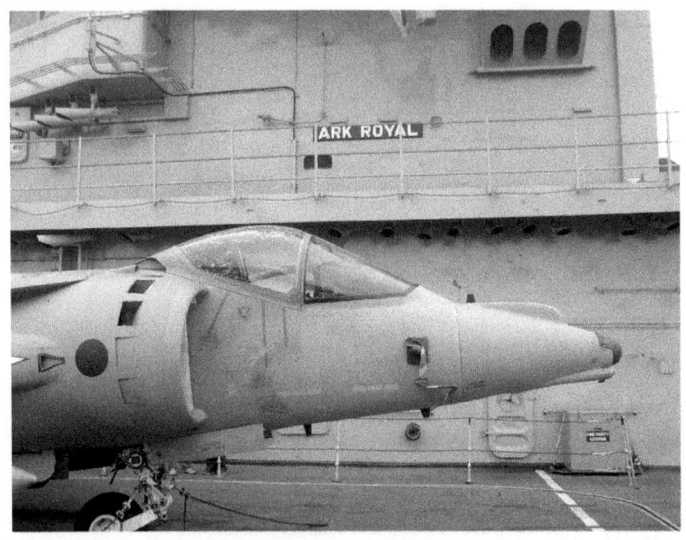

Harrier on deck.

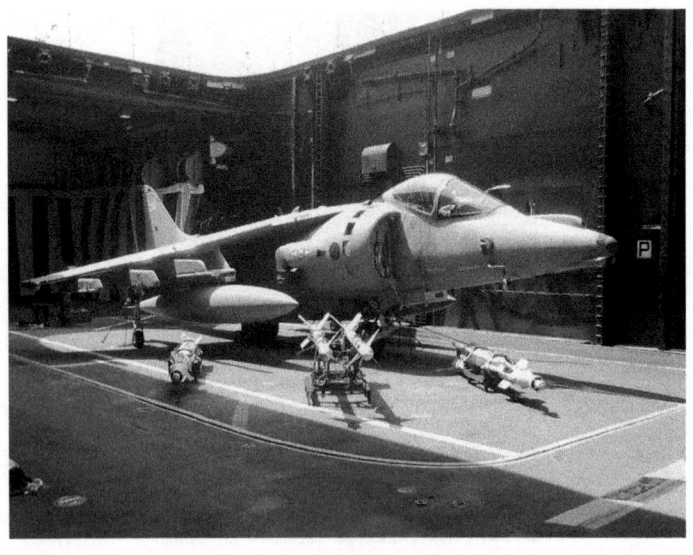

Harrier on lower deck.

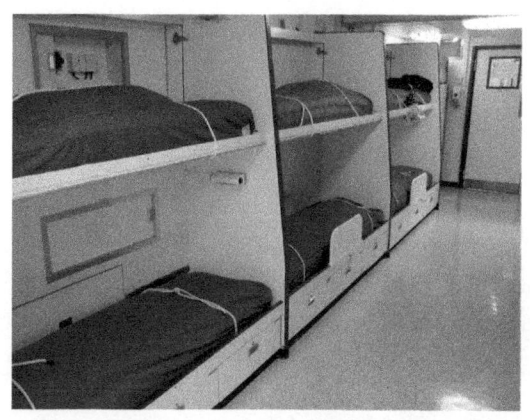

Hospital ward on ARK Royal.

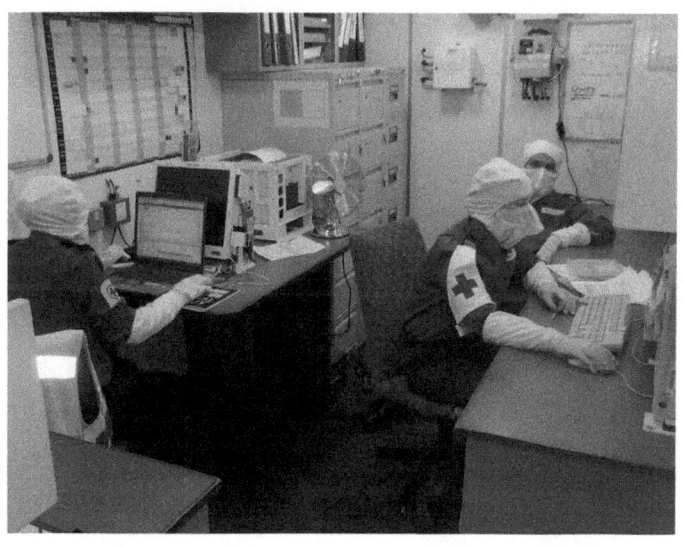

Medical team during 'action stations'.

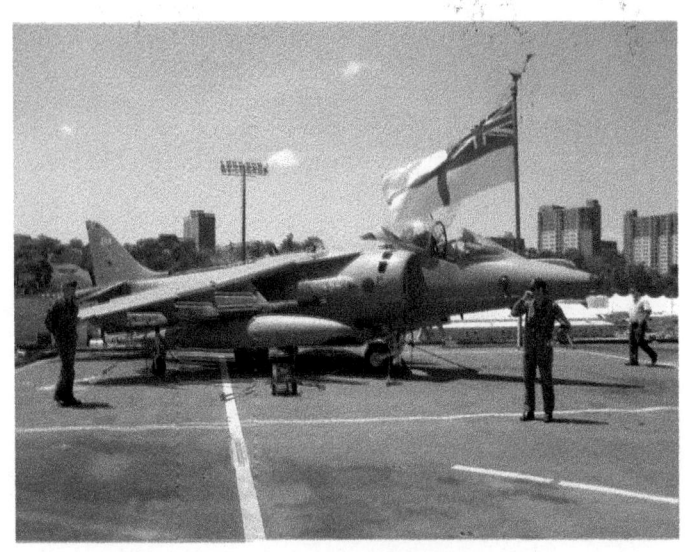

Open day on ARK in Halifax, Nova Scotia.

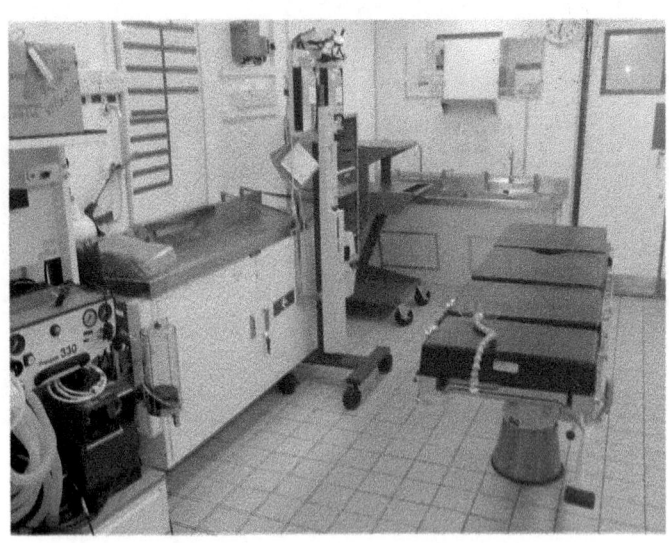

Operating theatre on ARK.

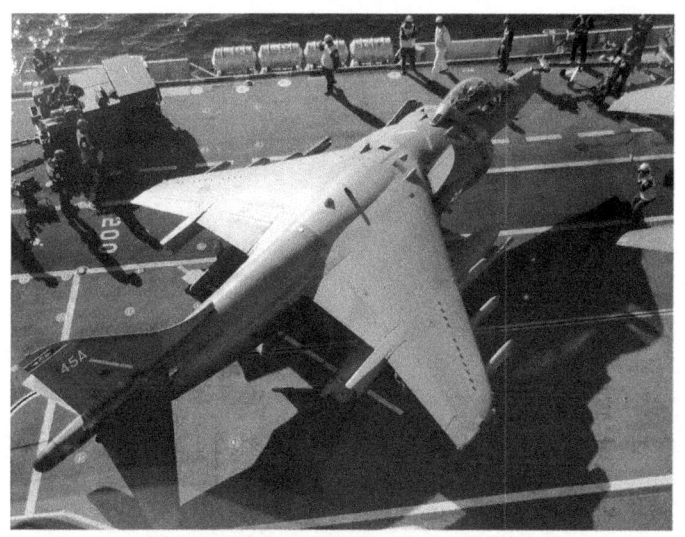

Ready for take-off.

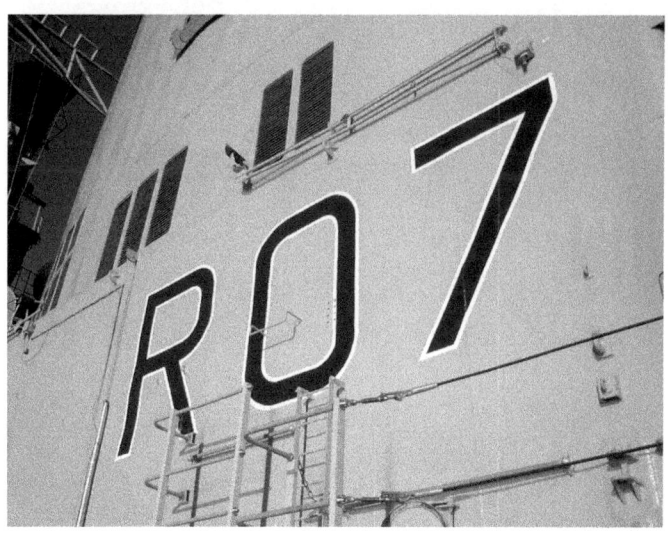

R07 Ark Royal's Identification.

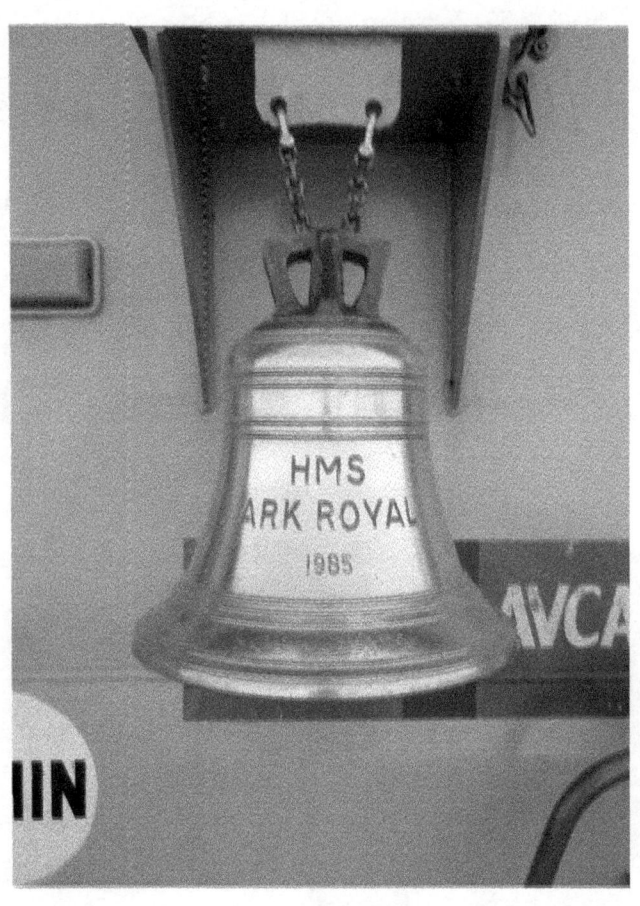

The ship's bell.

# 2004–2019: International Medical Repatriation Doctor

When I left the private practice in London in 2004, I was looking at ongoing work options. My interest in joining the Royal Navy was in the pipeline but I needed to have some income being generated. One day I saw an advert in the BMJ looking for medical repatriation flight doctors to go abroad and escort patients back home after either an illness or trauma that meant that they couldn't travel by themselves (Usually an insurance requirement). Having been a GP for over 25 years at this time and with my flying doctor experience in Australia, I quickly applied. I was soon invited to meet the medical director of the company who immediately offered me a position. The downside to this role was that it was all freelance with no guaranteed work, merely being available when a potential repatriation came up. Obviously whilst employed by the navy, my opportunities to do this job were restricted. Having said that, from 2004 until my retirement at the end of 2019, I had successfully repatriated 189 patients back from the far reaches of the world including New Zealand, Australia, various Caribbean islands, Mexico, India, S. Africa, Sri Lanka, the Philippines, Thailand, Indonesia, Iraq, Egypt, Israel, Brazil and Argentina (Over 50 countries in all).Some destinations were far less exciting such as the Canary Islands and Benidorm, especially when having to fly with Easy Jet or Ryanair but win some lose some. By far the commonest medical problem we've had was to repatriate those people who've had a heart attack. At least nowadays most patients get treated with a stent to open up narrowed coronary arteries whilst abroad so quite often they are healthier on the journey home than they were on the flight out. Having said that, thankfully, I have never had to administer CPR to anyone whilst flying at 38,000 feet.

My very first repatriation in 2004 was to fly out to Philadelphia, US, with a nurse colleague to collect two elderly sisters who had flown there to stay with family. During the car journey from the airport to the family's house, they were involved in a nasty road traffic accident. Both sustained multiple broken bones but nothing life-threatening. They spent the next 4–6 weeks either in the hospital or a private nursing home until they were fit enough to fly home. It was very reassuring having a nurse associate on my first repat, especially as there were two patients both requiring wheelchairs and it also helped with all the procedural aspects when transmitting through airports. I heard later that the medical costs alone in the US amounted to over £250,000 let alone that for the repatriation.

Doing this job has made me realise how many people travel abroad without adequate insurance. OK, until now anyone taken ill or injured within the EU can be treated by the EHIC arrangement but this generally only covers immediate basic investigations and care. No doubt this will change once the UK Brexit deal is formally completed. I do recall one irate chap who sustained a heart attack whilst in Italy, advised that he needed a heart bypass but told that he would have to wait until he returned to the UK to get this done. He couldn't appreciate that foreign hospitals only had to offer enough care to stabilise a medical condition.

I flew out to Turkey several years ago to collect a chap who'd had a heart attack but because he had no travel insurance, the hospital would not even consider inserting a coronary stent which is the usual treatment of choice. He did not have the financial resources to pay for this privately and in the end, had to appeal for crowdfunding from his hometown to cover the £10,000 that it cost to be in hospital and the repatriation.

One of my saddest repats was for a 26-year-old Sri Lankan woman who had been visiting relatives in Sri Lanka when she became extremely ill. She was already at this time on a waiting list for a heart and lung transplant but of course, donors for such transplants are few and far between. I was somewhat surprised that she had even been allowed to travel with such a condition. Even if she went ahead, she recalled how many of other patients she had met with similar problems, who had died shortly after surgery. So, she was left with a major predicament, to hold on and take her chances or go for surgery and risk an even more premature death. It was an uncomfortable flight back to the UK from Sri Lanka, all 11+ hours of it. I really thought I might lose her several times when her oxygen levels dipped quite low with the altitude but a bit of additional oxygen seemed to revive her (Normal blood oxygen saturation is 94–98). Normal for her was about 80% and she nearly died in the hospital abroad because the doctors tried to administer too much oxygen which nearly put her in respiratory failure. I was relieved to get back to the UK and successfully dropped her at home to her parents. I had a lovely e-mail a few weeks later saying how much I had helped her safely get home to her family. I didn't want to even contemplate what happened to her subsequently.

A lot of people seem to have acute psychiatric illnesses whilst on holiday. I didn't really like doing these repats as they can be quite unpredictable. In one such case, I had to go to Havana in Cuba where a 21-year-old lad had been celebrating his birthday with his mum. He had some form of acute psychiatric breakdown and was arrested by the local police after running down the tourist district completely naked. I caught up with him in a small tatty hospital a few days later where he was still tied by all four limbs to the bed and receiving regular intramuscular tranquillisers.

I guessed that he had probably sourced some dodgy weed or something similar. At this point, he didn't look in a fit enough state to fly back to the UK. I reviewed him the next day warning my team back in the UK that the repat could be 50:50. Actually, on review, he seemed much more relaxed and cooperative, helped no less by my insistence that the hospital staff remove his shackles and probably the fact that he'd had someone English to speak to. We decided to go for the repat and flew with KLM to London via Amsterdam as we needed an extra supply of oxygen on the long-haul flight. We were going to have a couple of hours in Schiphol airport before connecting to an ongoing flight to the UK. He insisted on being allowed to go and have a smoke. I thought this might at least calm him down. They had several glass rooms for this purpose within the terminal. They looked very unsavoury as one could only just see human outlines through the thick smog. His mum agreed to escort him and off they went. It seemed forever but they then announced the boarding details of our flight. But where was my patient? Mum came rushing back to our gate minus her son who she said had slipped out of the smoking room and disappeared. If anyone has tried to find a missing person in Schiphol airport, they will appreciate that it is a vast building with a number of walkways and gates in every direction. I rushed back and forth panicking as I'd lost my patient. Eventually, I saw him afar and caught up with him. As I patted him on the shoulder to let him know that it was me, he turned and gave me a whacking punch to the chest. Somehow, I manoeuvred him to our gate but not before he pushed an emergency alarm button setting other passengers off panicking. I gave him a large dose of Haloperidol as soon as we got on the plane and thankfully, he slept all the way home. I certainly earned my money on that trip.

Another psychiatric case was with a youngish chap who had been holidaying in a Red Sea resort with his wife and two children when he too had an acute psychotic episode. He was heavily sedated and aero-medded across to Cairo. I was sent to the hospital to bring him back home. I say hospital but the entrance to the facility was padlocked when I arrived with my driver/interpreter. We were led into a long dark corridor that had all the appearances of a prison block. My patient was actually in a cell with bars on the windows and door, the latter again heavily locked. I introduced myself. I don't think he had spoken English to anyone since his ordeal started a week or so earlier and he looked so pleased to see a fellow Brit. His cell was sparse. The staff had removed anything that could have been used as a noose, even his shoelaces and belt.

I couldn't help but notice the cockroaches scurrying across his cell floor and the dirty tin bucket in the corner which served as his toilet. Initial conversation didn't suggest any significant ongoing mental health issues, so I was happy to continue with the repat. We drove him straight to Cairo airport for the four-hour flight back to London without any problems and I didn't need to give him any other medication. It was very emotional seeing him reunited with his family after such an ordeal.

Another of my psychiatric repats was for a 17-year-old Indonesian lad who was doing a foundation degree course at Queens University in Belfast. The staff there were very concerned about his general behaviour, namely that he was stalking fellow students to the point of hiding behind hedges and walls often at night wearing camouflage clothing then keeping detailed notes of everyone's whereabouts. He had also been telling others how he had been trained in self-defence and martial arts and that he was quite capable of killing someone. The university's view was to get him back to Jakarta asap as he was only 17. I flew out to Belfast with a male psychiatric nurse and we escorted him back to Jakarta. It was a long 17-hour flight listening to my patient rambling on the whole time. Somehow, my psychiatric friend managed to sleep the whole journey.

Strangely, I then had another 17-year-old lad whom I repatriated back from Lusaka in Zambia. He had gone out there on a month's voluntary charity work experience from his Roman Catholic school in Ireland. Although the information we had been given by the staff at the camp was that he had had a psychiatric episode, when I first interviewed him there was no signs of this and it merely transpired that he couldn't cope having no TV, no mobile phone or use of a play station. And he'd only been there two days!

I had the chance to fly out to St Lucia and repatriate a chap of about 65 back to the UK. There was some suggestion of an alcohol problem but the main reason to send a doctor was because he had had a generalised seizure at his hotel. He had been investigated and was started on medication, so it all seemed a straightforward job. He was staying in a SAGA owned hotel so inevitably most of the residents were elderly and most it appeared were single. One of the residents came up to me and asked if I knew what SAGA stood for. I had no idea. "Sex and games in the afternoon" was his reply. My patient seemed quite normal and we got to the airport OK. Because we were flying back business class (Standard when doing a repatriation to give the patient a chance to sleep) I took him into the business lounge. I had to be very careful that he didn't slope off and get himself a G&T in view of his medical history, so I got him a large glass of orange juice. As we sat down to chat, to my embarrassment, he had a massive full-blown fit, ejecting his drink forcibly over several fellow-suited businessmen sitting nearby. Thankfully, it was only a short seizure and after some more medication, he remained well all the way back to the UK.

I've always enjoyed the long-haul flights when doing repatriations, especially when one is being treated to travelling in business class both ways. There was one occasion where a young Philippines ship steward had been taken ill in the Caribbean and had to be repatriated back to the Philippines. Another GP colleague flew out to the Caribbean and escorted him back to London where I would take over and fly with him back home. There was quite a long time between them landing at Heathrow and our onward flight to Manila, so my company booked us into a day room at an airport hotel for a rest before a 13–14-hour flight. It did not occur to me until sometime later what people in the hotel must have thought seeing an elderly man (Me) entering a luxury hotel with a 22-year-old Pilipino lad!

The flight was fine and uneventful. On landing in Manila, the lad's family were there to meet him with an ambulance and he was whisked off to a local hospital for further care. I now had two days in Manila with no constraints of a patient to restrict me. I'd been booked into the luxury Hyatt Regency hotel, so I was looking forward to relaxing and having a good look around.

I'd only been in the hotel for 3–4 hours when my company called me. "We have an urgent repatriation from Melbourne to London and as you're over that way, could you fly down there tomorrow and pick him up?" So much for my relaxing couple of days. I agreed, of course. My only concern was that I had only packed enough clothes for my original itinerary. Early the next morning, I flew the eight hours to Melbourne, met my second patient and within another 24 hours was on my way back to the UK. Another 24 hours in a plane. What a trip.

Another repat that caused a few raised eyebrows was when I escorted a very attractive 20-year-old girl back from Bali. She had been doing some volunteer work in a local school there and unfortunately, developed acute appendicitis followed by an epileptic seizure. The doctors operated on her successfully and started her on epileptic medication (Including quite potent anxiolytics and anti-depressants) which made her quite drowsy and wobbly on her feet to the point that I often had to support her. What none of us had been made aware of was the fact that she had had a number of previous seizures over the last year or so and not even informed her parents let alone the travel insurance company who if aware would probably not have forked out all this expense to get her home. I was acutely conscious throughout our trip home what other travellers were thinking about this elderly man with a very dishy young girl, especially as we were travelling in business class. Her clothing was what one would describe as 'Skimpy' and I'm sure many of them thought she was drunk. I felt like having a big banner over my shoulders saying, "Trust me, I'm a doctor." Perhaps they just thought that I was a dirty old man!

I've had a couple of repatriations which didn't go quite as expected.

On one occasion, I was on a BA 747 overnight flight down to Cape Town to pick up a chap who'd had a heart attack. I was nicely relaxed after dinner and ready to have a sleep. Then, over the tannoy came a call for any doctor to identify themselves. As much as one tries not to respond, there is no way one really can ignore such a call, so I pushed the call button and along came a cabin crew member. I was escorted downstairs (As I was in Club class) and taken to see an old chap who had collapsed in the aisle. A couple of nurses were already in attendance and they were very concerned that his BP and pulse were very low. He was semi-conscious. There wasn't much else any of us could do unless he needed defibrillating. I had to update the captain. He asked if he was safe to continue the flight to Cape Town. Bearing in mind that we were crossing the Sahara and that we still had several hours of flight time, I advised that we should get him landed as soon as possible. Our only option given our position was Lagos in Nigeria, not an ideal drop off point. However, the captain got all the clearances and permission to land which is what we did. As we descended, over the tannoy, the captain warned the passengers not to panic as he had to offload some aviation fuel otherwise, the 747 would be too heavy to land. It transpired that he jettisoned 30 tons of fuel at a cost of £30,000. We landed safely, offloaded our patient and then had to refuel! Four hours later than anticipated, we landed in Cape Town. I never did find out what happened to the old boy.

The second repatriation that didn't turn out quite as expected is when I flew out to Orlando to pick up another elderly man who'd had a heart attack but had had a stent fitted so was fit to return home in the UK. On the day I arrived, I went to see him and his wife at their villa and all seemed well and straightforward. I had a couple of days at my hotel until I had to pick them up for the drive to the airport. My taxi picked me up and we drove over to the patient's address. I got him settled into the taxi but as his wife got to the car, she collapsed on the drive. She went completely unconscious although still breathing. We were due on a flight to London in about four hours. What do we do? There was no way I could risk taking her on an eight-hour flight. We called 911 and within about ten minutes, we had a huge fire engine and a paramedic ambulance all lights and sirens blaring with eight emergency service personnel arrive. She was promptly piled into the ambulance and thoroughly examined. I was told that they would have to take her to A&E due to her poor observations. That was our return flight scuppered. We all trundled off to A&E and after further investigations, I learnt that she too had had a heart attack and would have to stay in the hospital a few days. Thank God, we weren't on the flight when this all happened. I then had the dilemma that I could still in theory take my original patient home but he refused as understandably he didn't want to leave his wife in the hospital alone. I called my office back in the UK and with their agreement, caught the next flight back to London alone (But at least in Business class!)

My scariest repatriation was when I was asked to fly out to Erbil in the Kurdistan region of northern Iraq to pick up an ex-Army bomb disposal expert who had been clearing old minefields for the oil and gas companies but had sustained a heart attack. At that time (2012) the area was considered a safe destination until it became the ISIS capital a couple of years later. There were no UK airlines flying there then so I had to go with Lufthansa via Frankfurt. It was quite apparent on the Frankfurt-Erbil flight that this was not your normal family holiday destination. All the passengers were men of a certain demeanour. I guessed most were either in the oil and gas industry or security. On arrival in Erbil, I was amazed at the modern state-of-the-art airport terminal, obviously funded by the west. I waited for ages in the baggage hall for my medical kit to arrive as did a couple of dozen other travellers but no sign of it. We eventually found out from the baggage handlers that our bags had not been loaded onto the plane in Frankfurt. So, I'm in a dodgy country in the Middle East supposedly to assess a patient's fitness to fly but without any kit to examine him with. They informed us that the bags would be delivered the following afternoon but as I was due to fly out again the next day, I asked them to keep my bag in Frankfurt so that at least I could collect it for the return flight to London.

I had been informed that I would be met in the arrival's hall by a couple of private security guards. Sure enough, these guys stood out like a sore thumb, 6'4" tall, tanned, built like wrestlers, wearing pale blue matching polo shirts with little logos sewn on. And each had a pistol holster dangling off their belts.

We drove off out of the airport but not before they picked up their guns from the main gate. I was taken to a very fortified accommodation compound where I met my patient, having to explain that I hadn't got any medical equipment. However, he was so keen to get home in the UK that he said to go on. I naturally had to clear this with my boss back home but from what I'd seen of the country so far, I didn't really want to stay any longer than was necessary. The two hulks then dropped me off at my hotel which was also heavily fortified. The guards at the gate thoroughly searched the car, looking underneath with mirrors. They even had sniffer dogs. I had to go through a scanner and my one and only small hand luggage was searched before I could even get through the hotel lobby. Then at the reception, the most amazing sight. As I checked in, other guests were arriving and handing over their pistols and semi-automatic rifles to desk staff in exchange for getting a cloak tag. I ate at the hotel that night but that was an uncomfortable experience as I was the only white Caucasian in the restaurant. All the others were wearing traditional full Arab attire.

I was glad when morning arrived. My hulks pitched up as arranged, we collected my patient and headed back to the airport. There was a long queue at the security barriers to the airport as everyone had to hand in their guns again. The flight to Frankfurt was uneventful. On arrival, we went over to the baggage handling office to collect my medical kit only to be told that they had inadvertently forwarded it on to Erbil.

Heaven knows what I would have done had my patient been unwell during the trip home.

Sepsis is a potentially life-threatening condition caused by the body's response to an infection. The body normally releases chemicals into the bloodstream to fight an infection. Sepsis occurs when the body's response to these chemicals is out of balance, triggering changes that can damage multiple organ systems.

I repatriated two young men back home after suffering from severe near-death sepsis. The first was a 19-year-old Australian man who was crewing on a private yacht in the Mediterranean. He sustained quite a minor graze to one of his shins, likely from some coral. Within a day or so, the area became very inflamed and swollen. He soon became feverish and generally unwell. He was admitted into a hospital in Nice where sepsis was diagnosed. He developed multi-organ failure such that he was put on a ventilator and received renal dialysis for over a month. His parents were flown over from their home in Hobart, Tasmania, as their son was given less than a 50% chance of survival. At this point, his parents looked into paying for a private air ambulance to take him home but were quoted £400,000! This sounds an awful amount but one has to bear in mind that it would probably involve a specialist Lear jet with extra crew, ITU doctors and nurses. Miraculously, he did recover and after a few more weeks recovering, I escorted him and his parents back to Tasmania. At this time, he was still unable to walk and had lost some four stones in weight.

The second patient with sepsis was a 29-year-old backpacker in New Zealand. He was found unconscious by a fellow traveller in a hostel. On admission to the hospital, he was diagnosed with Meningococcal septicaemia which also triggered the multi-organ failure. He too required two weeks on a ventilator and luckily recovered. That was a long flight back to the UK. The only consolation on this occasion was that this patient was staying only an hour away from where my daughter lived near Auckland so I did get the chance to meet up with her for a couple of days.

During my time working as a flight doctor, the vast majority of repatriations were conducted on commercial airlines. However, there were occasions when this would not be a practical option as for example, if a patient needed a stretcher or had to fly at low altitude for a medical reason. In this case, we used Beechcraft King Air twin prop aircraft, just like the ones that were used by the Flying Doctor Service in Australia. These had adapted cargo doors that could enable a full-size stretcher to be loaded.

For a while, these were complemented by a Lear jet. These were quite amazing to fly in but equipped with a stretcher and loads of medical equipment, not the glamorous leather seating or well-stocked bar as such a craft would normally be endowed. The main advantage with these was their speed (500 mph+). On several occasions, we flew to the south of France and Portugal and being able to land in much smaller provincial airfields, we could do the whole repatriation in a day.

I thoroughly enjoyed my time as a repatriation doctor. I got to visit numerous countries all around the world, stay in nice hotels, travelling business class and meet some lovely people who were universally really a pleasure to be with. I always found it remarkable what a close relationship one could build up in such a short space of time and I feel thrilled having been able to help so many people get back home after quite a traumatic ordeal.

Over the years, what this role has shown me more than anything is the importance of reliable and effective travel health insurance. After all, just a few pounds could save an ill person £1000s in costs.

# 2018: Time to Start Winding Down

I formally left the Royal Navy on 04 April 2012 after an extremely interesting and enjoyable eight years in service. I would have continued but 58 years old was the formal retirement age. The last phase of my varied medical career would be as a civilian medical practitioner (CMP) a GP but still within the military environment. For the first three years of this, I worked at the Defence College of Police training at Southwark Park just outside Portsmouth. This is where much of the D-Day invasion was planned by Churchill, Anthony Eden and Eisenhower and where the original D-Day wall map remains. Following this, I chose to work variable periods as a locum doctor and mainly for army practices across Hampshire, Wiltshire and Dorset, so that I could still continue doing my repatriation work.

By 2018, I felt that I was ready to start considering retirement as the demands of continuous professional training was getting harder and harder due to the lack of a firm work base and I did not feel that I could return to the NHS after so many years. At the end of 2019, I stopped work completely. I now have more time to visit my daughter and her family in Auckland, New Zealand, although it'll be hard having to pay for my own ticket after going out there several times on all expenses paid repatriations. My son who is married to Kaley with two beautiful daughters, Daisy and Tilly, is a little closer near Ipswich, Suffolk so we see them as often as we can. When I first considered general practice in the late 1970s, I thought that it would mean working in the same practice throughout one's career. Most of the GPs I came into contact with tended to stay in one practice until they either died or reached a ripe old age, some even into their 70s. It was almost a taboo to consider moving practices as it seemed to be as if the GP didn't have the guts to see it through. Although unwritten at that time, the old fashion view of a GP was that of a family man with a wife at home who could answer the phone when the doctor was out and this was indeed the case when I first started which obviously had an impact on family life. Only with the advent of pagers and then mobile phones did this make being on call a little easier. I remember our first portable practice phone; a huge Motorola 6800X with a corded hand piece and a battery the size of a brick. Even this didn't solve any of our problems since barely half of our rural practice area had adequate signal coverage.

It was in 1998 that I decided it was time to move on from my NHS practice, eight years after getting divorced and trying to pursue my dream to go and work in Australia. A few people thought that I was mad to leave a secure, well-paid job with the guarantee of a decent pension at the end of it all. The trouble was it was not much fun being a single 44-year-old doctor in a rural practice where GMC rules prohibit any personal liaisons with patients. Could I stay in the same job for another 20 or more years? To check that I wasn't developing some psychological problem or going mad making me take such major life-changing decisions, I arranged to see a very good psychiatrist friend for advice. He had recently lost his wife to cancer, so he too was in a state of flux about his future. We had a long chat and he suggested that I write down all the good reasons to leave and go to Australia and all the reasons not to. This was a very interesting exercise. I was most concerned that my children would think badly of me going away but to maintain contact I bought them a fax machine (How technology has changed since) and sent them letters several times a week. I had also been bought a VHS video player by my work colleagues on leaving the practice, and with this, I could post mini-cassettes home for them to watch. In addition to their trip over to WA, I went home on several occasions and we had holidays away. My former GP partners soon found a replacement partner and I don't even think that most of the patients I'd looked after for all those years even realised that I had gone.

In the end, the positives outran the negatives and that spurred me on to go ahead.

This move was the biggest life change I had ever had but as it turned out, I have experienced new worlds and adventures I'd never dreamt of. I do sometimes wonder how some of my old colleagues are getting on, 40 years or more sitting at the same desk.

If I had my time all again, would I do it all like this? I would certainly encourage other doctors to take some chances and explore differing career opportunities as 40 years is a long time. Then they too could write some fascinating stories as I hope you have been reading.

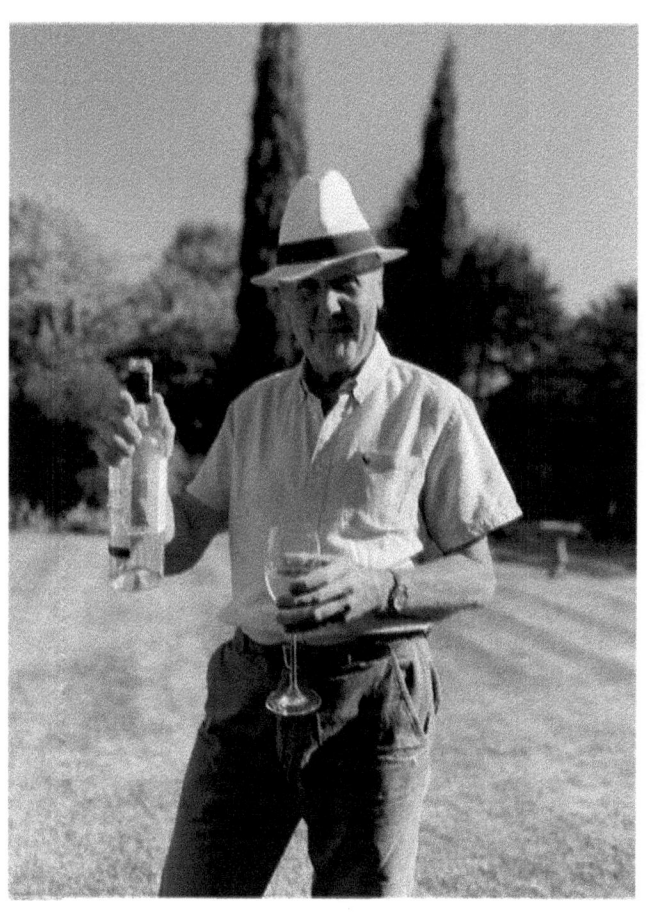

Peter Fowler

Ingram Content Group UK Ltd.
Milton Keynes UK
UKHW021514220623
423876UK00009B/153